Track and Field Self-Guided Workouts: Motivation and Activities

Mark Stanbrough, Ph.D.

Copyright © 2020 Roho Publishing.

All rights reserved. Printed in the United States

ISBN:978-1-945469-24-4

Roho Publishing
4040 Graphic Arts Road
Emporia, KS 66801

ABOUT ROHO PUBLISHING

When Kip Keino defeated Jim Ryun in the 1968 Olympic Games at 1500 meters, he credited the win to "Roho." Roho is the Swahili word for spirit demonstrated through extraordinary strength and courage. The type of courage and strength that can be summoned up from deep within that will allow you to meet your goals and overcome the challenges in life. Roho Publishing focuses on the spirit of sport and is designed to inspire, encourage, motivate and teach valuable life lessons.

DEDICATION

To all the coaches who make track and field fun. Your creative and positive attitude coupled with your passion towards track and field helps create a lifelong commitment for athletes to enjoy physical activity. The enjoyment received by your athletes has created lasting positive memories of track and field as well as offered tremendous positive benefits physically, psychologically, and socially. You make a difference in developing not only the physical components, but also the heart and minds of athletes.

ACKNOWLEDGEMENTS

To my family who have supported my passion for the greatest sport in the world—track and field. My wife, Wendy, has supported my endeavors in track and field as an athlete, coach, official and fan.

To my three daughters: Bethany, Leslie, Jenna, who have enjoyed participating in track and field and have remained die-hard track and field fans.

To Jenna, whose talents in developing this book have been invaluable. Her creative talents have been displayed in her artistic work involved in the layout, diagrams, covers and reviews

TABLE OF CONTENTS

Chapter 1	High Jump Games	1
Chapter 2	Long Jump Games	4
Chapter 3	Triple Jump Games	6
Chapter 4	Pole Vault Games	9
Chapter 5	Jump Games	11
Chapter 6	Shot Put Games	15
Chapter 7	Discus Games	18
Chapter 8	Javelin Games	20
Chapter 9	Throws Games	22
Chapter 10	Sprints Games	26
Chapter 11	Hurdles Games	33
Chapter 12	Distance Games	35
Chapter 13	Relay Games	42
Chapter 14	Motivational Stories	44
	References	75
	About the Author	76

INDEX

High Jump Games
High Jump Obstacle Course 1
Weave 1
Timed Figure Eight 1
Circle Gears 1
Circle Run-Simon Says 2
Time the J 2
Jump and Reach 2
Pop Weave 3
Shoe Kick 3
Limber Lower Now 3

Long Jump Games
River Leap 4
1 Step, 2 Step, 3 Step, 4 4
Standing Long Jump 4
Ancient Long Jump 4
Froggin' It 5

Triple Jump Games
Triple Jump Skip 6
Triple Jump Hopscotch 6
Jump Even 6
Triple Jump Rhythm 7
How Far Can You Triple Jump? 7
Leaps and Bounds 7
Lame Chicken 8
Distance Skip 8
Speed Triple Jump Bounding 8
One Stride Hurdle Hops 8

Pole Vault Games
Pole Run Agility Race 9
Pole Vault Sprint 9
Pole Vault Gymnastics 9
Pole Vault Abs 10
Pole Vault Strength Circuit 10

Jump Games
Frog Jumping 11
Leg Match with Partner 11
Banana Jumping Olympics 11
Jumping Bag of Balls 11
Indy 500 12
As If 12
Rope Skipping 13
Luck of the Draw Jumps 13
Jumping Popcorn 14

Shot Put Games
Shot Bowling Bash 15
Sponge Shot Put 15
Move It Back 15
On the Line 16
Towel Tally 16
Bean Bag Block 16
In the Hoop 17
Yarn Ball Toss 17
Thrower's Golf 17

Discus Games
Line Turn 18
Hoop Frisbee Throw 18
Rubber Chicken Throw 18
Flying Hoops 19
Flinging Square 19
Discus Freeze 19
Flinging Golf 19

Javelin Games
Noodle Target Throwing 20
Jamaica Javelin 20
Javelin Pentathlon 20
Javelin Acceleration 21
Javelin Snowball 21

Throws Games
Water Balloon Toss 22
Throwing Simon Says 22
Knee Throw 22
Overhead Backwards Throw 22
Hole in One 23
Throwers Trail 23
Luck of the Draw Throws 23
Medicine Ball Duathlon 24

Sprints Games
Armless Challenge 26
Calculating Stride Length 26
Spin and Start 26
Starting Ladder 27
Bean Bag Start 27
Ah Race 27
Cheetahs, Deer, and Elephants 28
Visualization Run 28
Stride Predictor 28
Sprinter's Pentathlon 29

Hurdles Games
Bricks and Sticks...33
Pizza Box Hurdle...33
Hurdle Mobility..33
Obstacle Course Hurdling.................................34
Dice Hurdling..374

Distance Games
Digital Scavenger Hunt..35
Sport Scenarios...35
Card War...36
Run and Pose..36
Dice Distance Running..36
Prediction Runs...37
Make-It-Take-It Intervals.....................................37
Scream Team..37
Runner's Pentathlon..38

Relay Games
Run and Get Back..42
Banana Relay..42
Wear the Shirt...43

Motivational Moments in Track and Field
Roger Bannister..45
Bob Beamon..46
Cliff Cushman...47
Raymond Ewry..48
Harrison Dillard..49
Rafer Johnson...50
Eric Liddell...51
Joe Kovacs...52
Aries Merritt..53
Edwin Moses...54
Dan O' Brien..55
Al Oerter..56
Steve Prefontaine...57
Derek Redmond...58
Louis Zamperini...59
Gretel Bergmann..60
Joan Benoit Samuelson.......................................61
Fanny Blankers-Koen..62
Michelle Carter...63
Alice Coachman...64
Gail Devers..65
Lolo Jones..66
Jackie Joyner-Kersee...67
Chaunté Lowe..68
Sandi Morris...69
Louise Ritter...70
Ana Fidelia Quirot...71
Betty Robinson...72
Brianna Rollins...73
Wilma Rudolph..74

PREFACE

Track and Field athletes are disciplined and committed. They desire to be active, but the challenge is how to stay active when you have to stay at home, work out by yourself and have limited equipment and facilities. *Track and Field Self-Guided Workouts: Motivation and Activities* contains multiple ideas, activities and games that can be used to create enjoyable and productive practice sessions that athletes can do alone, without a team and structured environment. It also includes motivational stories of track and field athletes who overcame hardship and diversity to succeed.

The numerous track and field games help teach the fundamentals and focus on skills required to become a more complete track and field athlete. The games are particularly useful for beginning and intermediate athletes and can be adapted to accommodate more traditional training with experienced athletes. The exercises are designed to challenge athletes and keep them active, motivated and thoroughly involved. The games can be competitive and fun to play and they can be easily adapted to different ages and abilities. Athletes respond favorably to activities in which they are excited and enthused about. The track and field activities provided in this book are designed to create and continue an enthusiastic and positive attitude.

It is not the intent of this book to give technical advice on "how to perform" the event correctly. Nor is it the intent to supply training programs and plans for athletes. The intent is to supply fun games that have specific objectives to develop athletes. *Track and Field Self-Guided Workouts: Motivation and Activities* combines fun with skill instruction and practice. The games are designed to utilize different approaches to track and field events while maximizing the development of physical skills.

This book is organized into different chapters. An activity that appears in one of the event-specific sections may be able to be used or modified for use in other events as well.

ORGANIZATION

The games have been organized in an easy-to-understand format as described below.

Objective: Consider a game's objectives to determine if the game fits your specific needs.

Description: This section supplies the directions in how to set up and run the activity effectively. Dimensions are provided only as general guidelines and should be adjusted to the ability level of athletes. In some games a scoring system has been provided to add an element of competition to the game. It should be clearly understood that the ultimate aim of each game is for athletes to challenge themselves to achieve a higher standard of performance.

Variations: These suggestions provide possible modification and adaptations of the games to offer more variety. The variations also may be used to adjust the difficulty and conditioning involved in the activity. Many of the variations allow the more naturally athletic or competitive athletes to enjoy play, while not exposing the less competitive athlete's weakness. You will have to adapt to meet the conditions and environment that you have.

Equipment: Most activities and games in this book have been designed to use a minimal amount of equipment and are easy to set up. Cones, balls, and ropes are some of the most common equipment items the games call for. You may have to substitute whatever items, objects or markers you may have.

SAFETY

Participation in track and field carries an inherent risk of injury. Minimize the risk by setting up the playing area with safety in mind, emphasizing safety, and making modifications as needed. Visualize how you want the game to progress and if the game does not conform to expectations, stop the activity and make adjustments.

HIGH JUMP

High Jump Obstacle Course
Objective: To integrate jumping rhythm, scissors jumping, and curve running

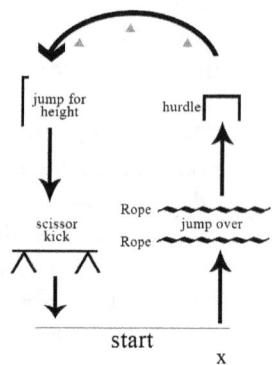

Description: Set up an obstacle course in a circular pattern with different types of jumps. You will navigate the course to see how fast you can complete the obstacle course. If possible, include a curve in the course to simulate the running approach, a scissors jump over a low object, a pop-up over a cone or low object, a low hurdle or object, a horizontal jump (such as jumping over two ropes) and something to jump and reach for.

Variations: (1) Complete the event for time. (2) Run the course multiple times to try to better your time. (3) Rate your technical skills on a scale of 1-10 on each jump.

Equipment: Cones, tape, or line to mark curve, ropes, small cones and crossbar, low hurdles

Weave
Objective: To practice running curved patterns involved in the high jump

Description: Set up a course of small cones or objects in a slalom pattern. Run the slalom course by weaving in and out of the cones and returning back to the starting line. Once you return to the starting line, rest, and repeat. For a left-hand approach, start on the left side of the cone/object, and for a right-hand approach, start on the right side.

Variations: (1) Run for time. (2) Run multiple times without stopping. (3) Run for a certain time and see how far you can get.

Equipment: Small cones or objects to run around

Timed Figure Eight
Objective: To develop the ability to run a fast curve approach

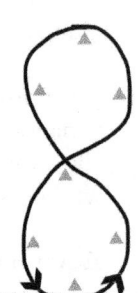

Description: Use cones or small objects to mark a 20-meter course. Set the objects in a figure eight pattern. You will run a figure eight to complete the course. Emphasize running tall and leaning into the curve. Time yourself to see how fast you can run the figure eight course.

Variations: (1) Run the course for time. (2) Run at least three times and see if you can improve your time. (3) Run for a certain time and see how far you can get.

Equipment: Cones or objects to run around, stopwatch

Circle Gears
Objective: To develop the rhythm and speed on a curve approach

Description: Set up a circle approximately 10 meters in diameter with small cones or objects. If you approach from the right side, you will run a counterclockwise circle around the objects. If you approach from the left side, you will run a clockwise circle around the objects. During the run, you will make gear changes. The speeds will be on a scale of 1-5, with 1st gear being slow and 5th being very fast. Start in "1" gear and run the circle. Lean into the curve on the run so your body weight is on the inside of the curve. After a lap, pick it up to gear "2." After one more lap, run a "3" speed for a lap and follow that with one lap at a "4" speed. The last lap is a "5" speed. Recover for a designated time period. Continue for a designated number of rounds.

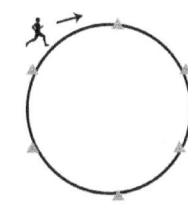

Variations: (1) Time to see how fast you can run the circle for one lap. (2) Extend each gear to two laps. (3) Alternate back and forth between gears (i.e., three to two to four to three to five). (5) Randomly pick your goals speeds.

Equipment: Cones or small objects, stopwatch

Circle Run-Simon Says
Objectives: To practice running the high jump curve

Description: Set up a circle approximately 10 meters in diameter with small cones or objects. If you approach from the right side, you will run a counterclockwise circle, if you approach from the left side, you will run a clockwise approach. Have a partner at a different location set up a similar course. Using telecommunications, decide who will go first. Partner 1 starts to run the circle. After 30 seconds, partner 2 indicates an activity by saying "Simon says do bounding." Partner 1 continues around the circle bounding. After 15-30 seconds, partner 2 changes the activity by saying something similar to "Simon says take three steps and pop-up." Partner 1 continue to run the curve and partner 2 calls out activities. However, if partner 2 does not say "Simon says" then partner 1 should continue the previous activity. If either athlete changes the activity when "Simon" did not say to, you must exit to the inside of the circle and jog in a clockwise direction until "Simon says" to do another activity and then you may re-enter the game. Continue for a designated period of time and then change partners running the curve.

Variations: Here are some recommended activities to do on the circle: (1) bounding, (2) change direction, (3) speed up, (4) high knees, (5) three steps and pop-up, (6) left leg jumping, (7) right leg jumping, (8) hopping on both feet, (9) Change or add your own.

Bonus Variation: Have multiple people on call or teleconference. Involve multiple athletes and trade off being "Simon."

Equipment: Cones or small objects to form a circle

Time the J
Objective: To practice approach speed

Description: Mark an area where the mat would be and where the standard closest to your take-off would be. Mark where you start for your takeoff approach. Mark where 20 meters past your takeoff approach would be. Run your full approach. The goal is to focus on your rhythm and increase speed with each step of the approach. Run 20 meters past the takeoff spot. Time from the first movement to the 20-meter spot.

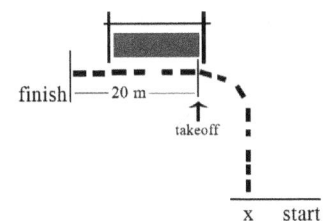

Variations: (1) Repeat by trying to beat your time.

Equipment: Area marked where start, takeoff position and 20 meters from takeoff position would be, stopwatch

Jump and Reach
Objective: To test vertical jump

Description: On a wall, measure your standing height from the end of your fingertip when you reach as high as you can with both feet entirely on the ground. Then measure the maximal standing vertical jump by jumping as high as you can and touching the wall. If you put a little chalk on your fingertips, it will be easier to mark it. Determine the difference between the standing reach and maximal vertical jump to calculate your vertical jump.

Variations: (1) Take the best of three trials on the maximal vertical jump. (2) Add up the three vertical jumps. (3) Come back periodically and see if you improve. **Bonus Variation:** (1) Communicate with your teammates and compare your vertical jumps. (2) Make teams and compete against each other by adding your scores up.

Equipment: Tape measure, chalk

Pop Weave
Objective: To practice running curved patterns and the take-off

Description: Set up a course of small cones or objects in a slalom course. Run the slalom course weaving in and out of the cones. When you pass near the cones, simulate the high jump plant by laying back in a plant position and performing a pop-up in the air. Do a pop-up in the air on every other cone. This allows you to jump on the same curve as your take-off approach. When the last cone is reached, go around the cone and return weaving in and out of the cones doing pop-ups. Once you return to the starting line, rest and repeat. Continue for a certain time period or until you have run through the cones a certain number of times.

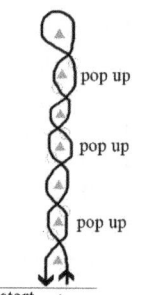

Variations: (1) Jump as high as you can on each pop-up. (2) Place different height cones or objects to jump over.

Equipment: Small cones

Shoe Kick
Objective: To take off using a scissor kick

Description: Untie and loosen your shoe on your take-off foot. Take two to three steps on a curve, plant your take-off foot and perform a scissor kick. Drive your inside leg up forcefully and powerfully and attempt to kick your shoe off your foot as far as you can. To complete the scissor kick, land with both feet on the ground.

Variations: (1) This can be done without a pit. Use a marked line to scissor kick over and land on your feet. (2) Measure how far the shoe can be kicked. (3) See how high the shoe can be kicked.

Equipment: Line to scissor kick over

Limbo Lower Now
Objective: To increase back flexibility for the high jump

Description: Find a broom stick or an item such as a pool noodle to use as a bar. Have someone hold or prop the bar up on obstacles. You will limbo under the bar. For the starting height, set the bar height so you can be successful. Use correct limbo technique. You must go under the bar by walking on your feet while keeping the back arched. You are "out" when you fail to achieve a height.

Variations: (1) Athletes get three attempts at a height before they are out. (2) Challenge a family member.
Bonus Variation: Telecommunicate with your teammates. Measure the starting height so everyone starts at the same height. Go one at a time. Put on some limbo music in the background!

Equipment: Something to use as a bar

LONG JUMP

River Leap
Objective: To develop dynamic coordination and rhythm

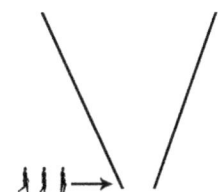

Description: Stretch out two ropes on the ground. Use the ropes to form a single large "V". The space between the two ropes is the river. With a short 1-2 step approach, leap over the river. Start leaping at the narrow part of the river and progress to leaping wider parts. Focus on the take-off with one foot and landing with two feet while bending the knees.

Variations: (1) Pretend there are crocodiles in the river and one must clear the gators!

Equipment: Two ropes

1 Step, 2 Step, 3 Step, 4
Objective: To practice short approaches

Description: Find a soft surface to run and jump on and mark a takeoff point to represent the take-off board. Take a jump off of a one-step approach. Record your distance. Then jump off a two-step approach and record your distance. Continue with a three-step approach, followed by a four-step approach and jump. Add up the distance for the total of jumps.

Variations: (1) Measure from where you actually take off instead of the designated takeoff mark. (2) Take multiple attempts at each approach length.

Equipment: Soft surface to land on, recording sheet

Standing Long Jump
Objective: To develop power by performing a standing long jump

Description: Mark a take-off point. Place your toes as close as possible to the starting line. Perform a standing long jump. Measure from the take-off line to where your back heel (on foot that lands closest to take-off line) lands. Perform a designated number of times.

Variations: (1) Add each jump to obtain a cumulative distance.

Equipment: Tape measure, Recording sheet

Ancient Long Jump
Objective: To experience a historical long jumping method

Description: In ancient times, a long jumper carried a weight in each hand. He would swing these weights as he ran down the runway and as he jumped, he would bring the weights forward to help throw him into the landing pit. This was designed to increase the distance of the jump. Place a weight of approximately one to two pounds in each hand and practice taking standing long jumps onto a soft surface and bring the weights forward during the jump. Remain holding on to the weights at all times. Compare the weighted jumps to the regular jumps. Do you feel the weights gave you an advantage? Note that it is now illegal in track and field to carry the weights.

Variations: (1) Take multiple jumps without the weights and measure the distance. Was there any difference between the lengths of the jumps with the weights and without the weights?

Equipment: Soft landing surface, tape measure, small weights or objects (1-2 pounds) to hold in hands

Froggin' It

Objective: To develop power in the jumping legs

Description: From a starting line, perform a "frog jump," a two-foot forward hop. The landing point becomes the starting line for your next jump. Repeat for a designated distance or period of time.

Variations: (1) Continued for a designated distance. (2). Continue for a designated time. (2) Alternate legs for one-leg jumping.

Equipment: None needed

TRIPLE JUMP

Triple Jump Skip
Objective: To develop the triple jump rhythm

Description: Have two people hold the ends of a skipping rope as the rope turns. Start away from the rope and hop, step and jump towards the rope. The goal is to make it over/under the rope without disturbing the rhythm. Emphasize the importance of even rhythm and maintaining speed throughout the jump. Continue for a designated number of times.

Variations: Use other jumping activities such as: (1) bounding, (2) right leg hop, (3) left leg hop, (4) skip, (5) two-foot hop, (6) Use as an individual activity turning your own jump rope.

Equipment: Long jump rope to be used for skipping

Triple Jump Hopscotch
Objectives: To develop dynamic balance, coordination, and rhythm required for the triple jump

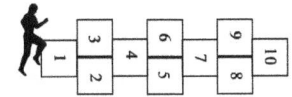

Description: Draw a hopscotch grid with 10 numbered boxes. Line up in front of the hopscotch grid. Toss a marker into square 1. Hop over square 1 and hop through all the other squares on one foot. At the end of the grid, turn around and jump all the way back on one foot, pausing to pick up the marker from square 1 and finish jumping back to the start. Next throw the marker into square 2 and go again and skip jumping in square 2. Continue to repeat until you have completed the hopscotch grid with the marker in every square. When there are two free squares side by side, land one foot in each square at the same time before continuing on one foot.

RULE: If you step into the square with the marker, touch any lines, or touch the ground with any body part other than the one foot, you must start again at square 1.

Variations: Try different hopping actions to go through the course: (1) left foot, (2) right foot, (3) alternate feet, (4) feet together, (5) hop, step, jump, (6) hopping backwards.

Equipment: Make your own hopscotch grid with chalk

Jump Even
Objective: To practice the rhythm of the triple jump phases

Description: Using ropes, cones, or markers, lay out a grid of three lines that get gradually farther apart from each other at one end. Within each grid is the phase landing area. At one end the three lines are close together, at the other end they are the furthest apart. The three lines at any one time should be equidistant to aid in making the three phases of the jump the same length. Start on the narrow end and try to jump in the phase areas using the triple jump sequence. For a greater challenge, continue moving down the grid where the landing phase areas are wider.

Variations: (1) Try clapping the rhythm you hear from the three phases. There should be no variation in time between phases. You could also chant "hop, step, jump" on each phase. (2) Score one point for each time you land in the proper phase landing area.

Equipment: Tape measure, rope or cones to mark grids

Triple Jump Rhythm
Objective: To practice the even rhythm of the triple jump phases

Description: Lay out a grid of three lanes consisting of three hula hoops, cones or objects laid end-to-end. In lane one, the three hoops are closer together, in lane two, the hoops become further apart and in lane three, the hoops are the furthest apart. One point is scored for every hoop you correctly jump into. Start in lane one, take a run-up of five meters or less, and complete a hop, step, and jump. After completing lane one, move into lane two, and then lane three. The score is recorded after every trial with the goal being to score the most points possible. Adjust the distance between hoops based upon the ability level.

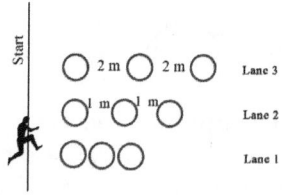

Variations: (1) Add a bonus point if all three grids are correctly hit.

Equipment: Tape measure, hula hoops, cones, or small objects, recording sheet

How Far Can You Triple Jump?
Objective: To have fun practicing the standing triple jump to see how far one can go

Description: You will compete in three different triple jumps and tally the total of all three. Place a line down to represent the take-off board. The first jump will be a standing triple jump from the take-off line. The measurement will be taken from where you take off (toe of front foot) to where you land (heel of foot closest to take-off point). The second triple jump is a two-step approach and jump from the take-off point. In the third jump, perform a four-step triple jump, taking off at your take-off mark and jumping as far as you can. After you have jumped all three jumps, add your total distance.

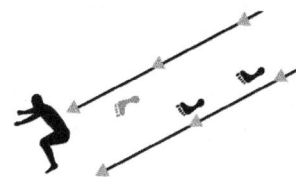

Variations: (1) Emphasize jumping and take the measurement from where you take-off, not from the take-off line. (2) Compete on virtual teams and add up the individual scores for a team total.

Equipment: Soft surface, tape measure, recording sheet

Leaps and Bounds
Objective: To have fun practicing bounding drills

Description: Mark out a 10-meter zone and a 30-meter zone. You will have three sets of bounding drills to complete for time.
- alternate single leg bounding for 30 meters
- alternate speed bounding for 30 meters
- double leg bounding for 10 meters

Record the times after each bounding exercise. Add up the three bounding drill times for a cumulative time.

Variations: (1) Conduct as a virtual team competition, with other jumpers playing from another location. Telecommunicate, or text each other your distances, adding up the individual times for team total. (2) Increase or decrease the bounding distance. (3) Bound and sprint. (4) Hurdle bounding.

Equipment: Markers, stopwatch, recording sheet

Lame Chicken
Objectives: To develop power and rhythm in jumping

Description: Place 10 popsicle sticks, or any type of stick, rod, or rope on the ground, spaced approximately one yard apart, in an even row. You must triple jump over the sticks by hopping over the first stick, stepping over the second and jumping over the third. Once you have completed the jump, begin again with the hop. After triple jumping over the 10 sticks, pick up the 10th stick and triple jump back to the start over the remaining nine. Once back to the start, begin jumping over nine sticks. This continues until all the sticks are picked up. If you touch the other foot to the ground or touch any stick, you must start over. You will not be able to complete all three phases on some jumps, depending on the number of sticks remaining.

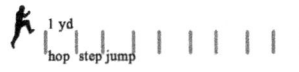

Variations: (1) Jump for time.

Equipment: Popsicle sticks, or rope

Distance Skip
Objective: To develop power and rhythm in jumping

Description: Skip for distance. Skipping for five skips and the distance is measured. Progress to skipping for 10 skips and measure the distance. Progress to skipping for 15 skips and measure the distance. Add up the total distance skipped.

Variations: (1) If possible, skip on a football field and use the yard lines to help determine distance or mark distance on the jumping field. (2) Instead of measuring, start the next skip set where the previous one ended.

Equipment: Tape measure

Speed Triple Jump Bounding
Objectives: To develop power and rhythm in jumping

Description: Use cones to mark a distance 10 meters apart. Time as you triple jump over a 10-meter distance. As you become advanced, move the distance up to 20 meters apart and then 30 meters.
Variations: Use jumping activities as repetitive hops: (1) left, left, left, (2) right, right, right, (3) alternate legs, (4) double leg hops, (5) bounding.

Equipment: Cones, watch

One Stride Hurdle Hops
Objective: To learn the explosion required on the final jump

Description: Line up six hurdles, cones or obstacles approximately three to four feet apart. Keep the obstacles low to begin with. Stand one stride away from the first obstacle and take one stride forward, bringing both legs together and squat with the arms behind the back and the knees bent about 90 degrees. Throw the arms forward and jump off both feet over the hurdle. Upon landing, take one stride forward and complete the same thing going over all six hurdles. Walk back and repeat for the desired number of repetitions.

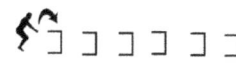

Variations: (1) Start with one to two hurdles then increase the number of hurdles. (2) As you more comfortable hurdling, focus on exploding over the hurdle and taking one step to explode over the next hurdle. (3) Time how long it takes to complete the hurdle circuit.

Equipment: Obstacles to represent hurdles

POLE VAULT

Pole Run Agility Race
Objective: To carry the pole and practice speed and rhythm in the approach

Description: Find something to use, such as a broom handle or a pool noodle to simulate a pole. Carry the pole practicing speed and rhythm in your approach. Set up a mini-hurdle agility course of 10 mini-hurdles (you may use small objects for this) about three meters apart from each other over a 40-meter distance. Start standing up (like one would in the pole vault), carry the pole, and race over the 10 mini-hurdles. When you become comfortable over the hurdles, you can increase the speed of the run. Eventually, you will sprint the course for time. This activity will increase your confidence to carry the pole.

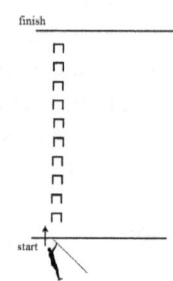

Variations: (1) Sprint a designated number of times trying to beat the previous best time. (2) Increase the number of mini hurdles with the hurdles closer together. (3) Increase the distance of the run. (4) Sprint over the hurdles without carrying a pole. (5) Time the difference between running with a pole and without a pole.

Equipment: Broomstick, pool noodle or something that simulates pole, mini hurdles or cones or small obstacles, stopwatch

Pole Vault Sprint
Objective: To carry the pole and practice speed in the approach

Description: Lay out a starting line and finish line 30 meters apart. Find something to use such as a broom handle or a pool noodle to simulate a pole. Race carrying a pole to practice speed in your approach. Sprint 30 meters holding the pole and using correct form. The time will start on your first move and will end when your body crosses the 30-meter finish line. Emphasize running through the line.

Variations: (1) Sprint the course a designated number of times, trying to beat your previous time. (2) Make the running distance shorter or longer (20 meters, 40 meters, 60 meters). (3) Time the difference between running with a pole and without a pole.

Equipment: Stopwatch, broomstick handle or pool noodle—something to simulate pole

Pole Vault Gymnastics
Objective: To perform gymnastic drills related to pole vaulting

Description: Use a soft field, carpet, or area with mats. Perform different gymnastic drills and score yourself. The scoring is similar to a gymnastics meet, with 10 being the highest score one can get and 1 being the lowest. The scores of all the drills are added for a total point score. The activities to be performed are:
- Back extension rolls
- Somersault, tuck jump, straddle jump in that order
- Handstand push-ups

Variations: (1) Add different activities. (2) Perform each activity individually and try to improve your score. (3) Pick the activities you want to do. They can be different from the list, as long as they are pole vault focused.

Equipment: Recording sheet, soft field, carpet, or mats

Pole Vault Abs

Objective: To strengthen the core while practicing pole vault techniques

Description: Perform various abdominal exercises specifically related to pole vaulting.

Exercises:
- Lie on the ground with the drive knee bent and arms above the head. Using only the abdominal muscles and keeping the drive knee in front of the other leg, swing up to a vertical position with the legs straight above the body and feet flexed.
- Lie on a bench starting with the legs straight in the air. Hold on to the bench above our head and slowly lower the feet down to the bench.
- Lie on a bench starting with the feet down, only using the ab muscles to swing the legs up to vertical with the feet flexed. See how fast you can get to vertical.

Variations: (1) Time each exercise and repeat to see if you can improve your time. (2) Compete against a member of your family or a teammate virtually to see who has the fastest time. (3) Make a circuit by completing each exercise as fast as possible

Equipment: Bench, stopwatch

Pole Vault Strength Circuit

Objective: To get stronger doing exercises that relate to the pole vault

Description: Hold your hands together with arms straight out in front of the body. Step onto a box with your right foot, drive your right knee and jump up onto the box, then stepping back off with the right leg. Then step on the box with your left leg, drive your left knee and jump onto the box, then step back off with the left leg. This is done with each leg five times.

Sit on the box and stand up on one foot driving the other knee and switch. Do this on each leg five times. Place one foot on the box and step out with the other foot in front of them. Perform five split leg squats, jumping if you can. The lead knee simulates the drive knee while pole vaulting, and if you choose to do the arms over head, this simulates strong straight arms at the take-off

Variations: (1) Perform the circuit with a weight. (2) Start with a light weight, then increase the weight. (3) Start with a low box and increase the height. (4) Do each exercise separately and time it. (5) Perform the circuit holding the weight above the head. (6) Emphasize proper technique.

Equipment: Various weights, boxes of different sizes, stopwatch

JUMPS

Frog Jumping
Objectives: To develop power and rhythm in the legs

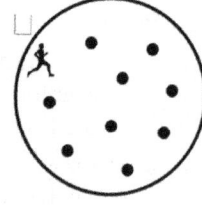

Description: Designate a jumping area. Start running around the jumping area. Every so often, get down like a frog and jump 3 times. This is a great warmup for jumpers.

Variations: Use a variety of jumping activities involving: (1) bounding, (2) one-foot hopping, (3) backwards jumping.

Equipment: Cones to mark the playing area

Leg Match with Partner
Objectives: To develop power and rhythm in jumping

Description: Partner up with another athlete via telecommunications. Delegate one partner as #1 and the other as #2. You will both simultaneously jump up and down five times. On the sixth jump, extend one of your legs. If you both extend the same leg, athlete #1 gets one point. If you both extend opposite legs, athlete #2 gets a point. The first player to reach 10 wins.

Variations: 1) Use both of the legs to take off. (2) Use the right leg only for take-off. (3) Use left leg only for take-off. (4) Emphasize jumping high. (5) Alternate same leg, different leg for each player.

Equipment: None needed

Banana Jumping Olympics
Objectives: To develop power in jumping

Description: Designate a starting line and a finish line about 30 meters apart. You will need a banana and will compete a series of series of different activities will holding the banana. Here are some ideas.
- Hold the banana under your armpit and hop on one leg down and back.
- Place the banana between the knees and hop down and back.

Once you have finished your activities, you may eat the banana!

Note: It is not required to eat the banana. It is often mushy by the time the activity is over.

Variations: (1) Use your own ideas and add a few variations to the list.

Equipment: Banana

Jumping Bag of Balls
Objectives: To develop power and strength in the legs

Description: Designate an area. Spread numerous balls or objects around the area. These balls or obstacles should be of different sizes and weights such as tennis balls, volleyballs, basketballs, footballs, and medicine balls. Start outside the playing boundary and run in to retrieve a ball. Pick up one ball or object and return it to a bag or box outside the circle by using a jumping mode such as hop back, big steps back, or jump back. Continue to retrieve balls until they are all deposited in the bag.

Variations: Use the following variations of jumping: (1) Two legs, (2) right leg only, (3) left leg only, (4) bound from right leg to left leg. (4) triple jump—hop, step, jump, (5) Assign points to different size balls.

Equipment: Bag of balls or obstacles of different sizes and weights such as tennis balls, volleyballs, basketball, football, medicine balls, cones to mark playing area.

Indy 500
Objectives: To develop power in jumping

Description: Designate a loop course. Give yourself a car name—Porsche, Ferrari, etc. Label index cards from 1 to 7. Shuffle the cards and place upside down by the start. Run around a designated loop. Your car can have problems with a related jumping activity to perform. After the first lap, as you begin every lap you will draw a card with a number. At any point on the lap you may stop and perform the activity that corresponds with the number on your card.

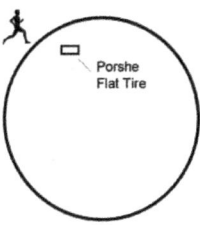

1. Flat tire- hop on one foot for 10 hops
2. Run out of gas- skip 10 times
3. Steering wheel- run zigzag for 10 meters
4. Rusty transmission three steps forward- two back 5- Front end mis-alignment- double hops for 10 hops
5. Turbo boost- bounding- 10 bounds
6. Yellow caution flag- tuck jumps vertically- 10

Variations: (1) Place signs around the course to indicate the activities to be performed. (2) Include a pit-stop for recovery.

Equipment: Cones to mark the loop

As If
Objectives: To develop strength and power in the legs

Description: Perform "as if" activities. Each activity should last 15-30 seconds with a brief (15-30 seconds) rest between the next activity.

Some sample activities for "As If":
- Run as though you were going to run around the world.
- Run as if Jason is chasing you with an axe.
- Walk forward as if you're walking in yogurt.
- Jump in place as if you are dunking a basketball.
- Reach up as if you are painting a ceiling.
- Step up as if you were climbing stadium steps to the top row of Yankee stadium.
- Jump on one leg as if you were popping popcorn.
- Bound as if you were a deer.
- Hop as if you were a frog in a frog-jumping contest. Shake your body as if you were a wet dog.

Variations: (1) Numerous activities can be substituted. (2) Have someone call out "as if" activities. (3). List "as if" activities on note cards and randomly draw them when it is time to perform a new activity.

Equipment: None needed

Rope Skipping

Objective: To develop power and rhythm in jumping

Description: Stand with feet parallel in the starting position, holding the skipping rope behind the body with both hands. To start, the rope is brought forward over the head and down in front of the body and you will hop over the rope. This cyclic process is repeated as many times as possible in 15 seconds. You should hop on both feet. Every touch of the ground by the rope is counted. Repeat for a designated number of rounds.

Variations: (1) Use the following modes of jumping: (1) Double leg hops, (2) right leg single, (3) left leg single, (4) hop-step-jump.

Bonus Variation: Form a team via telecommunications. Keep track of how many skips in a row you can achieve. The best result of each team member is scored for the total of the team. Repeat for a designated number of rounds.

Equipment: Jump rope

Luck of the Draw Jumps

Objective: To perform jumps based upon cards drawn

Description: You will need a deck of cards. Take a card without looking and then turn the card over. Return your card to the bottom of the pile. Perform the tasks designated on each individual card including the activity and the recovery. When finished with the tasks, draw a new card.

Luck of the Draw Jumps Activity	
Ace	Bound 30 meters
King	Jump on right leg for 20 meters
Queen	Jump on left leg for 20 meters
Jack	Jump off both feet for 20 meters
Joker	Triple Jump (hop, step, jump) for 20 meters
Odd number	Bound first 30 meters and jog 30 meters
Even number	Jog first 30 meters and bound last 30 meters

Luck of the Draw Jumping Recovery	
Heart	Rest 1 minute, return to start doing the same activity
Spade	Immediately jog back
Diamond	Rest 30 seconds, return to start doing the same activity
Club	Walk back to the start

Variations: (1) Take multiple cards at once and complete the tasks that are assigned. (2) Take one card for the activity and one card for the recovery.

Equipment: Deck of playing cards

Jumping Popcorn

Objective: To use a jumping activity simulating popcorn popping

Description: This activity imitates popcorn popping. Designate a playing area. Squat down to begin for the activity. When ready, jump up as high as you can, extending your arms overhead and shaking them vigorously to indicate the intensifying heat, then start jumping slowly on one leg. As the popcorn warms up, increase your speed. Just like popcorn kernels popping in all directions, you should change directions often. After 10- 15 seconds, squat down and prepares to repeat the activity.

Variations: Use a variety of jumping activities involving: (1) bounding, (2) two-foot hopping, (3) backwards jumping.

Equipment: None needed

SHOT PUT

Shot Bowling Bash
Objective: To work on the release out of the power position

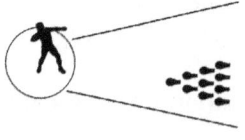

Description: Use a ball to simulate the shot. It could be a tennis ball, softball, baseball, etc. Make bowling pins by using two-liter plastic soda bottles filled with an inch of sand or other empty plastic containers. Set up the pin in the throwing area in the formation of bowling pins approximately 40 feet away from the throws release area. Throw from the power position and put the shot towards the pins. Remove the knocked over pins from the area. Then put a second time. Score as a bowling game. Reset the 10 bowling pins and continue to play a bowling game.

Variations: (1) Remove the down pins and keep throwing until all the pins have been knocked down. Keep track of the number of throws. (2) Move the throwing line back. (3) Throw from the full position.

Equipment: Bowling pins simulators, shot simulator such as softball or bean bag

Sponge Shot Put
Objectives: To work on throwing out of the power position

Description: Use a small dry sponge for a shot. Line up on the throwing line and put the sponge. Wherever the sponge lands is where you will throw again.

Variations: (1) Throw for a designated number of times. (2) Throw out of the discus power position. (3) Throw out of the javelin power position. (4) For fun on a warm day, throw a wet sponge. (5) Take full throws.

Equipment: Small dry sponges, bucket of water for hot days

Move It Back
Objective: To develop experience in moving backwards

Description: Many novice shot putters have difficulty with the glide in staying balanced while moving backward due to a lack of leg strength to execute the glide correctly. To get experience in moving backwards and to develop leg strength, try the following:

- Backwards running (timed for 20 meters)
- Backwards hopping on two feet (timed for 20 meters)
- Backwards jumping off drive leg (timed for 20 meters)
- Backwards lunges (timed for 20 meters)
- Backwards glides (timed for 20 meters)

Variations: (1) Add the total times. (2) Repeat and try to improve your times on each segment.

Equipment: Cones or markers to mark the 20-meter course

On the Line
Objective: To develop experience and control in the glide movement

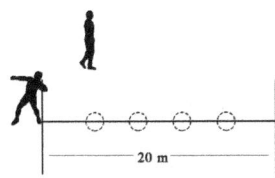

Description: Line up on a line. This could be a track line track, football field with marked lines, or any line you make. Begin from the shot put starting position, push off with the back leg and glide backwards with the goal of placing the heel of your foot and the toe of the front foot on the line. Freeze when you land and check your foot position. You receive one point for landing the front foot on the line and one additional point for landing the back foot touching the line. Continue to go down the line for 20 meters, scoring points for every foot touching the line. Continue for a designated time period.

Variations: (1) Time yourself for 20 meters down the line.

Equipment: Lines, cones

Towel Tally
Objective: To develop power gliding across the shot circle

Description: In the shot put glide technique, the initial momentum for the shot begins with a powerful backward thrust of the drive leg, which projects the thrower across the shot circle. This initial push-off is important because it increases the horizontal momentum of the shot; the stronger the drive, the more potential to throw further. The "towel drill" will help you improve your initial push-off. Begin in a starting position (facing the back of the circle). Place a towel 3 inches from the heel of your drive foot—the foot that's in contact with the ground and provides the force for the glide across the ring. As you perform a backward glide across the circle, push up and over the towel by driving your hips up and across the circle. You will score three points for gliding over the towel and one point for stepping on it. **Note:** This does not have to be done in the shot put ring, as there is not throwing involved.

Variations: (1) Increase the distance of the towel from your drive foot. (2) For every inch the towel is from the drive foot, score one point.

Equipment: Towel

Bean Bag Block
Objective: To practice throwing out of the power position

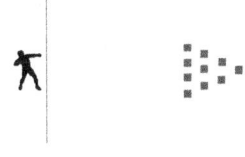

Description: Set up 10 cups or small similar objects in a pyramid formation approximately five meters from a throw line. Line up on the throw line with bean bags. Bean bags are thrown one at a time using the shot put technique from the power position, in an attempt to knock down the cups. When all the cups are knocked down, sprint to collect the bean bags and cups and then return back to the throw line. If all the cups are not knocked down, and you run out of bean bags, sprint to retrieve the bean bags and return with them to the throw line to throw again.

Variations: (1) Move the cup formation back to 10 meters and use the discus power position to initiate the throw. (2) Move the block formation back to 15 meters and use the javelin power position to throw.

Equipment: Blocks or cups to stack, bean bags

In the Hoop
Objective: To work on throwing out of the power position

Description: Design a throwing area with a throwing line and hula hoops or something similar to mark an area. The hoops should be placed one, two, and three meters away from the throwing line. You should have three bean bags. Throw from the power position of the shot put. After you have thrown all three bean bags, retrieve your bean bags.

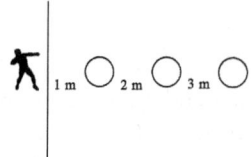

Variations: (1) Score one point for the first hoop, two points for the second hoop, and three points for the third hoop. (2) Throw in sequence with the first throw landing in the first target, the second throw landing in the second target, and third throw landing in the third target. Receive one point for landing the bean bag in the designated target. (3) Move the targets farther back. (4) Score points only if you throw properly out of the power position.

Equipment: Bean bags, hula hoops

Yarn Ball Toss
Objective: To practice throw release

Description: Hold a ball of yarn and stand on a throwing line. Hold onto the end of the strand of yarn with your non-throwing arm and put the yarn ball. How far does the yarn ball go? Measure the yarn from your hand to the spot where the yarn ball lands. Throw three times and to try to improve the distance each time.

Variations: (1) Throw from the power position. (2) Use a full throw.

Equipment: Ball of yarn, measuring tape

Thrower's Golf
Objective: To throw the shot and attempt to reach a target in the least number of throws

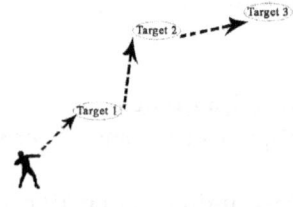

Description: Establish a course with cones or other objects as targets (holes) spread out throughout the course. Attempt to reach the target by shot putting bean bags. You must throw using the shot put technique. The first throw occurs from a throw line (the tee) and you throw to the next target (cone or object representing the next hole). After throwing, you will throw again from where the bean bag lands. Score the total number of throws to each target. The lower the score, the better.

Variations: (1) Vary the distance of the targets. (2) Increase or decrease the size of the targets. (3) Use tennis balls instead of bean bags.

Equipment: Objects to create targets (such as cones, towels, chairs), bean bags or tennis balls

DISCUS

Line Turn
Objective: To improve movement through the ring

Description: Line up on the lane lines of the track or make a line. Use correct discus technique and turn on these lines slowly, maintaining good balance as you turn and trying to stay on the line. Stress staying on the balls of the feet to allow the turns to be done rhythmically. You can increase the speed on turns as you become more competent.

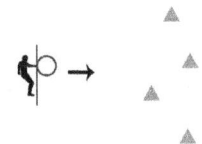

Variations: (1) Turn on the line for 20 meters and score a point for each foot that touches the line. (2) After each turn, freeze and re-establish balance and begin again. (3) Use a cone to experience the pull of an object while you go through turns.

Equipment: Marked line

Hoop Frisbee Throw
Objective: To work on the release in the discus

Description: Spread a number of hula hoops on the ground, or mark circles on the ground. Line up on the throwing line at five meters away from the target and have five throws to throw a frisbee, discus style into one of the hoops. Score one point for every frisbee thrown into a hoop if the throw demonstrates proper discus throwing technique.

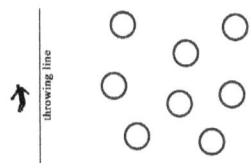

Variations: (1) Move the throwing line back a further distance. (2) Vary the game by assigning each hoop a different point value. (3) Add up the points you earn for five frisbee tosses.

Equipment: Hula hoops, frisbees

Rubber Chicken Throw
Objective: To work on the release

Description: How far can you throw a rubber chicken? You will use correct discus throwing form and throw a rubber chicken (or find anything that resembles) from the discus power position. Throw from the starting line and then run and retrieve. Throw three times with the total of each throw measured and recorded. The rubber chicken (or other item) will allow you to feel the pull of the discus movement as you sling it.

Variations: (1) As an alternative, throw a rubber cone.

Equipment: Rubber chicken, tape measure

Flying Hoops
Objective: To work on the release in the discus

Description: Set up cones or objects spread throughout a landing sector. Use hula hoops and use a discus style throw and attempt to throw the hoops over the cones. Score one point for every time they land a hoop over a cone.

Variations: (1) Start from a standing, power position throw. (2) Use a full throw. (3) Assign the cones a different point value.

Equipment: Cones, hula hoops

Flinging Square
Objective: To practice the power position of the discus

Description: Form a square with a bean bag at each corner. Start in one corner of the square with a bean bag. Assume the power position in the discus and fling to the next corner of the square using the discus style throwing method. The throws should go in a counterclockwise direction. Once you have thrown, go to the next corner of the square. Continue for a designated period of time. Once you have thrown four times, retrieve the bean bags to each corner of the square.

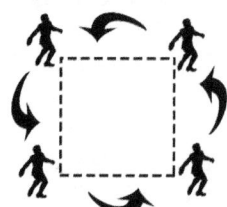

Variations: (1) Adjust the size of the square.

Equipment: Bean bags, cones, or something to mark the four corners

Discus Freeze
Objective: To focus on throwing out of the power position

Description: Designate a playing area. Run around the area. Approximately after 30 seconds, yell "freeze," or have someone yell "freeze." Assume the start of the discus throwing motion and hold this frozen power position. Check your form and readjust into a good position. Next, call "heat," which will melt your frozen position and then continue your throwing motion. Halfway through yell "freeze". After you freeze, check your form and readjust into a good position. Call "heat," which will melt your frozen position and then continue your throwing motion and get into the power position as you yell "freeze". Check your form. Call "heat" again and explode out of the power position and simulate the discus release. You are then free to start running again and repeat the process.

Variations: (1) Change the size of the playing area. (2) This could be done for all throwing events, including shot put and javelin.

Equipment: Cones to define playing area

Flinging Golf
Objective: To practice throwing from the power position

Description: Set up a course of cones or markers similar to a golf course. Designate a starting point and call that the first tee. Attempt to fling a hula hoop from the tee over the cone or marker in as few as tries as you can, out of the discus power position. Keep track of your own number of throws. Once successful, go on to the next hole.

Variations: (1) Creative athletes can assess a "par" for each hole. Determine par for each hole. (2) Lengthen the distance between holes.

Equipment: Hula hoops, cones or object

JAVELIN

Noodle Target Throwing
Objective: To focus on the javelin release

Description: Use pool noodles or insulation for hot water pipes. These should be approximately one meter long. You may wish to cover the center 10 centimeters with duct tape to serve as a grip. Line up on a designated throwing line. Assume the power position in javelin throwing and throw the makeshift javelin (using proper javelin technique) at a cone or object placed five meters from the throw line. Run and retrieve your throw and run it back to the throw line. One point is scored for every time you hit the target. Play for a pre-determined time limit.

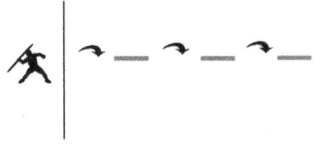

Variations: (1) Adjust the target distance of the cone to suit the distance that you can throw.

Equipment: Pool noodles, tape, markers

Jamaica Javelin
Objectives: To work on throwing out of the javelin power position

Description: Designate a starting throwing line and a finishing throwing line 40 meters apart. Use a pool noodle and stand behind the throwing line. Throw the noodle out of the power position and then sprint after it. Wherever it lands, pick it up and throw again out of the power position. Time how long it takes to throw past the finish line.

Variations: (1) Count the number of throws it takes to reach the finish line. (2) Extend the distance between the starting line and the finish line. (3) Play for a designated time and see how far you can throw.

Equipment: Pool noodle, stopwatch

Javelin Pentathlon
Objective: To improve throwing power in multiple activities

Description: Perform the following throws with the performances measured and recorded. Add up the five throws to get the total score. Adapt to whatever equipment you have and space available.

Overhead basketball throw
Standing overhead throw 1kg med ball
One handed – 1 kg med ball
Overhead shot put
Standing throw Pool noodle

Variations: (1) Measure each throw. (2) Take three trials of each throw, use the best of three.

Equipment: Basketball, 1kg med ball, shot puts, Turbo Javelins or any other useful and safe equipment

Javelin Acceleration
Objective: To focus accelerating all the way through the javelin approach

Description: Start at your take-off mark holding a pool noodle or something similar to simulate javelin. Use your full approach. The goal is to continue to accelerate all the way to the throw. If possible, have someone time you. It is a little more difficult to time yourself but possible. Your time should start with your first movement on the start to the final foot plant. You should not throw. The goal is to improve the acceleration.

Variations: (1) Try to improve your time. (2) Throw. (3) Time stops after you release.

Equipment: Stopwatch

Javelin Snowball
Objective: A fun activity during snowy days that focuses on the power position

Description: Every year, the Norway National Snowball throwing champs are conducted with kids and adults throwing softball sized snowballs over 80 meters. Make your own snowballs ranging from baseball to softball size. Or you can use a baseball or softball. Line up on the throwing line and throw for distance. Emphasis should be on the proper power position from a standing position.

Note 1: You are not throwing at other people. **Note 2:** You may use a baseball, softball, or tennis ball in place of a snowball.

Variations: (1) Take a full approach throw and throw from the throwing line. (2) Step off the distance and record in number of steps and try to better your throw.

Equipment: Snow, softball, baseball, or tennis ball

THROWS

Water Balloon Toss
Objectives: To practice correct technique of the throws

Description: Fill several balloons with water. Use correct form to throw the water balloon by shot, discus, or javelin technique.

Variations: (1) Use the discus throwing technique and throw the water balloons with two hands from the hip. (2) Use the javelin throwing technique and throw the balloons with two hands from high overhead.

Equipment: Water balloons

Throwing Simon Says
Objectives: To practice throwing events using shadow movements

Description: Start on a line without a throwing implement. You will perform shadow movements. Through telecommunications, a partner will be the leader (Simon). Simon will indicate a throwing activity by saying something like "Simon says, do discus throws from the power position." After 15-30 seconds, the leader (Simon) will change the activity by saying something similar to "Simon says glide across the ring as if throwing the shot." However, if the leader does not say "Simon says," then you should continue the previous activity. If you change the activity when "Simon" did not say to, you must jog in place for 30 seconds until "Simon says" to do another activity and then may re-enter the game. After a designated period of time, switch leaders.

Variations: Here are some recommended activities to do for throwers. You can change or add your own. (1) Power position throws for shot (2) Power position throws for discus (3) Power position throws for javelin (4) Shot put spins (5) Shot put glides (6) Discus rotation through the circle (7) Javelin cross overs

Equipment: None needed

Knee Throw
Objective: To practice throwing using proper upper body position

Description: Kneel on a mat, leans back (putting torque on the upper body) and heave a medicine ball (1kg) or other ball, using a two-handed overhead forward throw for maximum distance. After throwing, you should fall forward onto a mat with the follow through. Retrieve the ball. Record the best of three trials.

Variations: (1) Add up all three throws.

Equipment: Medicine ball, soft mats, tape measure, recording sheet

Overhead Backwards Throw
Objective: To use the legs in throwing backward for distance

Description: Stand with legs parallel, heels on the throwing line and back to the direction of the throw. The medicine ball (or other ball) is held down at arms' length with both hands. Squat down (placing a stretch on the thigh muscles) and quickly extend the legs, then the arms in order to heave the medicine ball backward over the head for maximum distance into the throwing area. After the throw, you may step backwards over the throwing line. Measure your distance.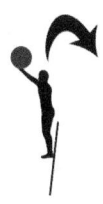

Variations: (1) Record the best measurement of the three trials. (2) Add up all three throws for and record total measurement.

Equipment: Medicine ball, tape measure, recording sheet

Hole in One
Objective: To practice throwing out of the power position

Description: Place a bean bag collecting bucket in the center of the playing area. Throw from around the circle, which is three meters from the bucket. Utilizing either the shot put, discus, or javelin technique, attempt to get a "hole in one" by throwing your bean bag in the bucket. Focus on throwing out of the power position and maintaining proper form. Retrieve the bean bags and repeat from a different spot on the circle. Play for a designated time or until a certain point value is reached.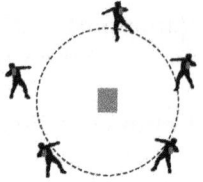

Variations: (1) Increase the diameter of the circle. (2) Use different throwing techniques such as shotput, discus and javelin.

Equipment: Bean bag, bucket for target

Thrower's Trail
Objective: To perform different activities as throwers go back and forth in serpentine style on the throwers trail

Description: Make three lines marked by cones or other objects and call them thrower trails. The trails will start at the starting line (trail head) and go to a cone that will be the turn-around point. Trail 1 begins at the far-left corner of area. Perform activities down and back on the trail and then move to the next trail. After you get to trail three, go to trail one. This is a continuous activity. As soon as you get back to the trailhead, move to the next trail and keep going. On each trail there, will be a specific activity to complete as you make your way down the trail.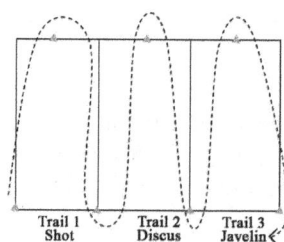

Trail 1: shot glide or spin
Trail 2: discus spin
Trail 3: javelin approach

Variations: (1) Vary the activities used on each trail. (2) Add an exercise zone at the end of each of the turnaround cones and perform a different exercise on each trail.

Equipment: Cones or something to mark the exercise stations

Luck of the Draw Throws
Objective: To perform throwing related activities based upon cards drawn

Description: You will need one deck of cards. Take a card without looking and then turn the card over. Remember your card. Return your card to the bottom of the pile. Perform the tasks designated on each individual card. When finished with the tasks, draw a new card.

Luck of the Draw Throws Activity	
Ace	10 med ball pounds into ground
King	10 shadow throws from shot power position
Queen	10 shadow throws from discus power position
Jack	10 shadow throws from javelin power position
Joker	10 shot glides
Odd number	10 discus spins
Even number	10 javelin cross overs

Luck of the Draw Throws Recovery	
Heart	Rest 1 minute
Spade	Jog 50 meters
Diamond	Rest 30 seconds
Club	Walk 50 meters and then jog back

Variations: (1) Perform the exercise on the card only and not the recovery. (2) Take multiple cards at once and complete the tasks that are assigned to them. (3) Take one card for the activity and one card for the recovery.

Equipment: Deck of playing cards

Medicine Ball Duathlon
Objective: To assess the development of throwing power

Description: You will compete in two throwing events. Points will be scored based upon the throwing performance. Record the points for each event and total the points at the conclusion. The goal is to score as many points as possible.

Standing Throw: Face forward with the medicine ball held overhead in two hands. Feet should be parallel and toeing the measuring line. Throw the ball for distance. A follow through step is allowed.

Three Step Throw: Start with both feet together in a stationary position. Take three steps forward with the medicine ball held overhead in two hands. Throw the ball for distance. A follow through step is allowed.

Light Medicine Ball:
Perform a standing throw with a medicine ball (men 2 kg, women 1.5 kg). Mark the point where the medicine ball lands. Measure and record the distance from the front foot (on release) to where the ball lands.

Heavy Medicine Ball:
Perform a standing throw with a medicine ball (men 3 kg, women 2 kg). Mark the point where the medicine ball lands. Measure and record the distance from the front foot (on release) to where the ball lands.

Variations: (1) Choose between either the light ball or heavy ball competition, depending upon the athlete level. (2) Perform both the light and heavy ball competition.

Equipment: 1.5 kg, 2 kg, and 3 kg med balls, 30-meter tape measure

Light Med Ball

Points	Standing Throw Distance (meters)	3 Step Throw Distance (meters)
1	3.00	4.50
2	4.50	6.00
3	6.00	7.50
4	7.50	9.00
5	9.00	10.50
6	10.50	12.00
7	12.00	13.50
8	13.50	15.00
9	15.00	16.50
10	16.00	17.50
11	17.00	18.50
12	18.00	19.50
13	19.00	20.50
14	20.00	21.50
15	21.00	22.50
16	22.00	23.50
17	23.00	24.50
18	24.00	25.50
19	25.00	26.75
20	26.00	28.00
21	27.00	28.75
22	28.00	29.50
23	29.00	30.25

Heavy Med Ball

Points	Standing Throw Distance (meters)	3 Step Throw Distance (meters)
1	2.00	2.75
2	3.25	4.00
3	4.50	5.25
4	5.75	6.50
5	7.00	7.75
6	8.25	9.00
7	9.50	10.25
8	10.75	11.50
9	12.00	12.75
10	13.00	14.00
11	14.00	15.25
12	15.00	16.50
13	16.00	17.75
14	16.75	18.50
15	17.50	19.25
16	18.25	20.00
17	19.00	20.75
18	19.75	21.50
19	20.50	22.25
20	21.25	23.00
21	22.00	23.75
22	22.75	24.50
23	23.50	25.25

SPRINTS

Armless Challenge
Objective: To focus attention on the use of the arms during running

Description: Identify an uphill area to safely sprint up. The first sprint up the hill is performed by holding your arms behind your back and running full speed up the hill. Record your time. Allow a sufficient amount of time to go back down the hill and recover. The second sprint is run with your normal sprinting arms. Compare the time between not using the arms and using the arms. Repeat the activity three to five times. Note the differences in comfort, power, and speed in armless running versus normal running.

Variations: (1) Restrain the arm swing by carrying two small cups, each filled halfway with water. (2) Try to balance tennis balls on big spoons in each hand as you sprint up the hill.

Equipment: Stopwatch, recording sheet

Calculating Stride Length
Objective: To examine the role of stride length in sprinting

Description:
Walking: Walk a normal pace over 100 meters and count the number of steps taken. To calculate stride length, divide 100 by the number of steps the athlete takes. For example, if you take 80 steps to cover the 100 meters, the stride length will be 100 meters divided by 80 which equals 1.25 meters per stride. Another way to measure stride length is to walk through a water puddle onto dry pavement and measure the heel-to-heel distance of the wet footprints.

Jogging: Jog over 100 meters and counts the number of steps taken. To calculate stride length, divide 100 by the number of steps taken. For example, if it takes 60 steps to cover the 100 meters, the stride length will be 100 meters divided by 60, which equals 1.67 meters per stride.

Sprinting: Sprint over 100 meters and counts the number of steps taken. To calculate stride length, divide 100 by the number of steps taken. For example, if it takes 40 steps to cover the 100 meters, the stride length will be 100 meters divided by 40, which equals 2.5 meters per stride.

Compare the stride length at different speeds. Stride length and stride frequency are the two major components of increasing speed and running faster. Increasing stride length is achieved by resistance training methods such as flexibility, plyometrics, weight training, uphill running, and pulling weighted objects.

Variations: Convert steps to mileage. (1) Walk for a designated period of time and count the steps. Multiply the number of steps by your stride length to determine how far you have walked. (2) Jog for a designated period of time and count the steps. Multiply the number of steps by your stride length to determine how far you have jogged. (3) Sprint for a designated period of time and count the steps. Multiply the number of steps by your stride length to determine how far you have sprinted.

Equipment: Tape measure, stopwatch

Spin and Start
Objective: To practice coming out of the starting position

Description: Jog slowly in a straight line. Periodically, jump in the air and turn around 180 degrees and immediately fall into a starting "set" position. This starting position is only held for 1-2 seconds before you will accelerate out of that position and sprint for 10 meters. After

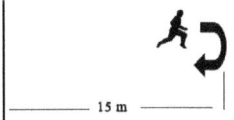

sprinting, begin jogging slowly again in a straight line. Recover before repeating the spin and start. Continue for a designated number of times.

Variations: (1) Assume the start "set" position for five seconds and then stand up and begin jogging (do not sprint out). (2) Go down into the "on your marks" position, hold it for three seconds, come into the "set" position, and hold for one second and then accelerate out of that position. (3) Come up to the set position and then start on your command.

Equipment: None needed

Starting Ladder
Objective: Working on the start and the first few steps out of the blocks

Description: Mark off 5 meters, 10 meters, 15 meters, 20 meters and 25 meters. Work on the start by coming out of the starting blocks (or without blocks if you do not have) on your command and running five meters at full speed. Run hard past the five-meter mark, as there is a tendency to slow down before the end. The second time out of the blocks, sprint for the first 10 meters. Progress to 15, then 20, then 25 meters.

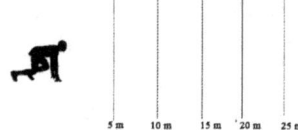

Variations: (1) Time yourself if possible (or have someone else time you). Run the starts again and try to beat your times. (2) Add up the times of all five starts and compare to other athletes.

Equipment: Starting blocks if possible, stopwatch, recording sheet

Bean Bag Start
Objective: To improve the arm action in the start out of the blocks

Description: Assume the starting position in the blocks. Place one bean bag, small stick, or object on top of the right hand and one bean bag or small stick on top of the left hand. Give yourself the set and "go" command. Drive the arms hard coming out of the blocks. The arm opposite the front step will fly forward vigorously throwing the bean bag forward. The arm opposite the back foot will vigorously throw the bean bag backwards. Take a couple of steps out of the blocks, stop, and returns to the blocks. Challenge yourself to see how far you can throw the beanbags.

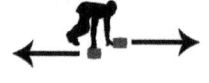

Variations: (1) Measure how far you can throw the bean bags. (2) Increase the number of steps you take after coming out of the blocks.

Equipment: Starting blocks, bean bags, small sticks, or small objects to throw

Ah Race
Objective: To see how far athletes can sprint while holding their breath

Description: Mark a running area with a marker placed every 10 meters up to 100 meters or run on a football field. Take one large inhalation. Begin running and yelling "Ahhhhhhhhhhh" running and continue yelling until you have to take a breath. That is round one. If you hit the end and are still "ahhhing," turn around and continues back. One point is awarded for every 10 meters you can run. Perform another round and see if you can better your performance. Continue for a designated number of rounds to see how many points can be scored.

Variations: (1) Mark off every 5 meters. **Bonus Variation:** (1) Compare yourself to teammates through telecommunication.

Equipment: Cones to mark every 10 meters

Cheetahs, Deer, and Elephants

Objective: To simulate running like different animals to experience what the changing speeds of fartlek feels like

Description: Spread out over the designated playing area. Start running around the area. You have numerous animals to imitate. If you call out "cheetah," you will sprint and imagine you are a cheetah. When "deer" is called out, run at a fast pace (but not all out), concentrating on good form imagining you are a deer running. When "horse" is called out, you will run at an easy pace. When "dog" is called out, you will jog. When "turtle" is called out, you will walk slowly. Call out both fast and slow animals to allow for both higher intensity running and recovery. This is an excellent activity for introducing fartlek training where you can feel the difference between changing speeds.

Variations: (1) Incorporate the use of different animals. (2) To progress to harder workouts, increase the length of time for faster animals. (3) To decrease the recovery time, allow less time for slower animals.

Equipment: None needed

Cheetahs, Deer, and Elephants	
Animal	Pace
Cheetah	Sprint
Deer	Fast Pace
Horse	Easy Pace Run
Elephant	Race Walk
Dog	Jog
Turtle	Walk slowly

Visualization Run

Objective: To enjoy visualizing a scenario while running

Description: Designate a running area. Run for a self-designated time and act out a dream. Below is a list of possible scenarios. While running, act out what the scenario might look like and feel like. For example: winning the Olympic Games, setting a 100-meter world record, or beating Usain Bolt. After a designated time period, allow a short recovery period and pick another dream to act out.

Possible visualizations:
- anchoring a winning 4 x 100 relay
- setting a new world record in the 200 meters
- upsetting an Olympic Champion
- winning the state championship
- outsprinting Usain Bolt
- setting a world record in the 100 meters
- anchoring a come-from-behind win in the 4 x 400 relay
- beating the best runners in the world at 400 meters

Equipment: None needed

Stride Predictor

Objective: To estimate the number of strides it takes to run to destinations

Description: Pick an object to sprint to, anywhere from approximately 50 to 400 meters away. The exact distance to the object does not need to be known. Before starting the run, predict how many strides it will take to run the designated distance to the object. Count every stride you take as you run to the object. Run in a normal stride length. When you arrive at the chosen destination, remember your total number of strides. Compare your predicted stride count to your actual stride count. Remember, you are on the honor system!

Variations: (1) Run a measured known distance, such as 100 meters, and count your steps.

Bonus Variation: (1) Challenge a friend via telecommunications. Run multiple times and tally the total difference at the end to see who was closest to their prediction.

Equipment: None needed

Sprinter's Pentathlon
Objective: To determine what kind of all-around sprinter you are in an event-scored decathlon style.

Description: You will do five runs: 300 meters, 100 meters, 200 meters, 50 meters, 400 meters, with 10-30 minutes recovery time between runs. Points are scored for each sprint based on the running time with the use of a decathlon scoring type chart. With an equal mix of different length sprints, this competition challenges you to determine how good of an all-around sprinter you are. You will run the 300 meters and find your time on scoring chart. Compare the time to the corresponding score on the scoring tables and record your score in points. Give yourself a certain amount of recovery time (15 minutes for workout, 20-30 minutes if you are using the sprinter's pentathlon as a competition). Start the next event, the 100 meters, and time. Find your time on the scoring chart and record the points off the scoring tables. Keep a running cumulative total. Continue the event by running 200 meters, 50 meters, and 400 meters. After the last event, calculate your total points.

Variations: (1) Use a long version of the Sprinter's Pentathlon by running 400-100-50-200-800. (2) Make it a family event. Compete against each other or on teams.

Equipment: Scoring chart, scoring tables, stopwatches.

Short Version Scoring Table

Points	300 meters	100 meters	200 meters	50 meters	400 meters
700	31.17	9.9	19.78	5.8	44.45
690	31.56	10.01	20.02	5.86	44.99
680	31.96	10.11	20.26	5.92	45.54
670	32.36	10.22	20.5	5.98	46.09
660	32.76	10.33	20.74	6.04	46.64
650	33.16	10.43	20.99	6.1	47.2
640	33.57	10.54	21.23	6.16	47.76
630	33.98	10.65	21.48	6.22	48.33
620	34.4	10.76	21.73	6.28	48.9
610	34.81	10.87	21.99	6.34	49.48
600	35.24	10.99	22.24	6.4	50.06
590	35.66	11.1	22.5	6.47	50.64
580	36.09	11.21	22.76	6.53	51.23
570	36.52	11.33	23.02	6.59	51.83
560	36	11.44	23.29	6.65	52.43
550	37.4	11.56	23.55	6.71	53.04
540	37.84	11.68	23.82	6.76	53.65
530	38.29	11.8	24.09	6.83	54.26
520	38.74	11.92	24.37	6.89	54.89
510	39.2	12.04	24.64	6.95	55.52
500	39.66	12.16	24.92	7.01	56.15

490	40.12	12.29	25.2	7.07	56.79
480	40.6	12.41	25.49	7.13	57.44
470	41.07	12.54	25.78	7.19	58.1
460	41.55	12.67	26.07	7.25	58.76
450	42.04	12.8	26.36	7.31	59.43
440	42.53	12.93	26.66	7.37	1:00.10
430	43.03	13.06	26.96	7.43	1:00.79
420	43.53	13.19	27.27	7.49	1:01.48
410	44.04	13.33	27.57	7.55	1:02.18
400	44.55	13.47	27.89	7.61	1:02.89
390	45.07	13.61	28.2	7.67	1:03.61
380	45.6	13.75	28.52	7.74	1:04.34
370	46.14	13.89	28.85	7.8	1:05.08
360	46.68	14.03	29.18	7.86	1:05.82
350	47.23	14.18	29.51	7.92	1:06.58
340	47.79	14.33	29.85	7.98	1:07.35
330	48.35	14.48	30.19	8.04	1:08.13
320	48.93	14.63	30.54	8.1	1:08.92
310	49.51	14.79	30.89	8.16	1:09.73
300	50.1	14.94	31.25	8.22	1:10.54
290	50.71	15.11	31.62	8.31	1:11.37
280	51.32	15.27	31.99	8.37	1:12.22
270	51.95	15.43	32.37	8.43	1:13.08
260	52.58	15.6	32.75	8.49	1:13.96
250	53.23	15.78	33.15	8.55	1:14.85
240	53.89	15.95	33.55	8.64	1:15.76
230	54.57	16.13	33.96	8.7	1:16.70
220	55.26	16.32	34.38	8.76	1:17.65
210	55.97	16.51	34.8	8.82	1:18.62
200	56.69	16.7	35.24	8.88	1:19.62
190	57.43	16.9	35.69	8.94	1:20.64
180	58.2	17.1	36.15	9.00	1:21.69
170	58.98	17.31	36.63	9.06	1:22.77
160	59.79	17.52	37.12	9.12	1:23.88
150	60.62	17.74	37.62	9.18	1:25.03
140	61.48	17.97	38.14	9.24	1:26.21
130	62.37	18.21	38.68	9.3	1:27.44
120	63.3	18.46	39.25	9.36	1:28.72
110	64.26	18.71	39.83	9.42	1:30.05
100	65.28	18.98	40.44	9.48	1:31.45
90	66.34	19.27	41.09	9.54	1:32.91
80	67.46	19.57	41.77	9.6	1:34.46
70	68.66	19.88	42.49	9.67	1:36.11
60	69.95	20.23	43.27	9.73	1:37.88
50	71.35	20.6	44.12	9.79	1:39.81
40	72.89	21.01	45.06	9.84	1:41.94
30	74.65	21.48	46.12	9.9	1:44.36
20	76.73	22.03	47.38	9.96	1:47.23
10	79.45	22.76	49.03	10.02	1:50.97

Long Version Scoring Table

Points	400 meters	100 meters	50 meters	200 meters	800 meters
700	44.45	9.9	5.8	19.78	1:46.8
690	44.99	10.01	5.86	20.02	1:47.8
680	45.54	10.11	5.92	20.26	1:48.9
670	46.09	10.22	5.98	20.5	1:49.9
660	46.64	10.33	6.04	20.74	1:50.9
650	47.2	10.43	6.1	20.99	1:52.0
640	47.76	10.54	6.16	21.23	1:53.1
630	48.33	10.65	6.22	21.48	1:54.1
620	48.9	10.76	6.28	21.73	1:55.2
610	49.48	10.87	6.34	21.99	1:56.3
600	50.06	10.99	6.4	22.24	1:57.4
590	50.64	11.1	6.47	22.5	1:58.5
580	51.23	11.21	6.53	22.76	1:59.6
570	51.83	11.33	6.59	23.02	2:00.8
560	52.43	11.44	6.65	23.29	2:01.9
550	53.04	11.56	6.71	23.55	2:03.1
540	53.65	11.68	6.76	23.82	2:04.2
530	54.26	11.8	6.83	24.09	2:05.4
520	54.89	11.92	6.89	24.37	2:06.6
510	55.52	12.04	6.95	24.64	2:07.8
500	56.15	12.16	7.01	24.92	2:09.0
490	56.79	12.29	7.07	25.2	2:10.2
480	57.44	12.41	7.13	25.49	2:11.4
470	58.1	12.54	7.19	25.78	2:12
460	58.76	12.67	7.25	26.07	2:13.9
450	59.43	12.8	7.31	26.36	2:15.2
440	1:00.1	12.93	7.37	26.66	2:16.6
430	1:00.8	13.06	7.43	26.96	2:17.8
420	1:01.5	13.19	7.49	27.27	2:19.1
410	1:02.2	13.33	7.55	27.57	2:20.4
400	1:02.9	13.47	7.61	27.89	2:21
390	1:03.6	13.61	7.67	28.2	2:23.1
380	1:04.3	13.75	7.74	28.52	2:24.5
370	1:05.1	13.89	7.8	28.85	2:25.9
360	1:05.8	14.03	7.86	29.18	2:27.3
350	1:06.6	14.18	7.92	29.51	2:28.7
340	1:07.4	14.33	7.98	29.85	2:30.2
330	1:08.1	14.48	8.04	30.19	2:31.7
320	1:08.9	14.63	8.1	30.54	2:33.2
310	1:09.7	14.79	8.16	30.89	2:34.7
300	1:10.5	14.94	8.22	31.25	2:36.3
290	1:11.4	15.11	8.31	31.62	2:37.8
280	1:12.2	15.27	8.37	31.99	2:39.4

270	1:13.1	15.43	8.43	32.37	2:41.1
260	1:14.0	15.6	8.49	32.75	2:42.7
250	1:14.8	15.78	8.55	33.15	2:44.4
240	1:15.8	15.95	8.64	33.55	2:46.2
230	1:16.7	16.13	8.7	33.96	2:47.9
220	1:17.6	16.32	8.76	34.38	2:49.7
210	1:18.6	16.51	8.82	34.8	2:51.6
200	1:19.6	16.7	8.88	35.24	2:53.5
190	1:20.6	16.9	8.94	35.69	2:55.4
180	1:21.7	17.1	9	36.15	2:57.4
170	1:22.8	17.31	9.06	36.63	2:59.4
160	1:23.9	17.52	9.12	37.12	3:01.5
150	1:25.0	17.74	9.18	37.62	3:03.7
140	1:26.2	17.97	9.24	38.14	3:06.0
130	1:27.4	18.21	9.3	38.68	3:08.3
120	1:28.7	18.46	9.36	39.25	3:10.7
110	1:30.1	18.71	9.42	39.83	3:13.2
100	1:31.5	18.98	9.48	40.44	3:15.9
90	1:32.9	19.27	9.54	41.09	3:18.6
80	1:34.5	19.57	9.6	41.77	3:21.6
70	1:36.1	19.88	9.67	42.49	3:24.7
60	1:37.9	20.23	9.73	43.27	3:28.1
50	1:39.8	20.6	9.79	44.12	3:31.7
40	1:41.9	21.01	9.84	45.06	3:35.8
30	1:44.4	21.48	9.9	46.12	3:40.3
20	1:47.2	22.03	9.96	47.38	3:45.8
10	1:51.0	22.76	10.02	49.03	3:52.9

HURDLES

Bricks and Sticks
Objective: To introduce beginners to the hurdles

Description: This activity can be used as an introductory drill before attempting to use real, full sized hurdles. It is based upon the 'bricks and sticks' approach of hurdling over a low height and gradually increase the height of the hurdle. The use of a yardstick, broomstick, or pool noodle balanced on blocks allows a gradual increase of the height by progressing to multiple wooden blocks. Spread out the jumping obstacles so that there is plenty of room to hurdle.

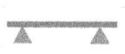

Variations: (1) Start with one hurdle and emphasize good form. (2) When you become comfortable with running over the "bricks and sticks," add multiple barriers. (3) Increase the distance between hurdles.

Equipment: Cones, crossbars

Pizza Box Hurdles
Objectives: To learn beginning hurdling skills and develop a rhythmic pattern

Description: Beginner hurdlers often think the hurdles are a jumping event and slow down and jump too high vertically over the obstacle. This activity allows the beginning athlete to run over an obstacle that is low to the ground and maintain sprint form. Set pizza boxes or other similarly sized objects on the ground about five meters apart. Sprint over the pizza boxes.

Variations: (1) Time yourself over the boxes. (2) Add pizza boxes on top of each other to make a higher hurdle height. (3) Focus on sprinting. (4) Jump over an actual pizza and eat it when done (don't step on it). (4) Order a pizza!

Equipment: Pizza box

Hurdle Mobility
Objectives: To improve flexibility and power

Description: Set up four to seven hurdles in a line close together (a couple of feet). If you do not have hurdles, find something to simulate hurdles. The hurdles should be set at an optimal height that allows you to stand astride the hurdle while standing on your toes. Maintain a tucked hip position and move the arms in conjunction with the legs. Step over each hurdle.

Variations: Try the following: (1) lead with left then right, (2) walkover— only one foot lands between each, (3) backward walkovers, (4) step-overs, (5) sideways step, (6) over-under (focus on hip flexors), (7) hold hands overhead or behind the head for advanced balance training, (8) hold a medicine ball.

Equipment: Hurdles or something to simulate hurdles.

Obstacle Course Hurdling

Objective: To work on hurdling over different obstacles and using different step patterns

Description: Develop a loop course with a total distance of approximately 100 meters long. One area will be the sprint area, one area will be designed for sprinting over hurdles (or other barriers) and one area will be designed as a slalom course to sprint around. Run for a designated number of loops or time.

Variations: (1) Time yourself.

Equipment: Low obstacles to jump over, low hurdles, cones for slalom

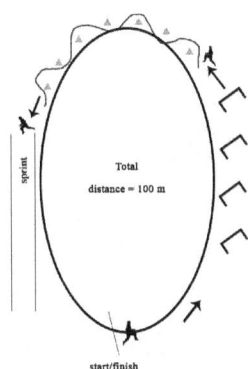

Dice Hurdling

Objective: To determine the number of hurdles to run based upon the roll of dice

Description: Roll one die to see how many hurdles you will run at one time. After you run, return to roll the die again to determine the next run.

Variations: (1) Roll 2 dice and add up the numbers and run over that number of hurdles (do not surpass a total of 10 hurdles).

Equipment: Dice, hurdles

DISTANCE

Digital Scavenger Hunt
Objective: To find items on a scavenger hunt by taking digital pictures

Description: Make a list of things you want to find on your digital scavenger hunt. Designate your running boundaries and a time to be back. Take a digital camera or a cell phone camera with you on your run. Take a picture of everything you find on your list.

Sample list of items to take pictures of:
Sign with letter "r" in it
Black Dog
Sign that says name of the town
Pinecone
Cow
Tractor (not a riding lawnmower)
Person riding a bike
Two birds in the same picture
Flowers in bloom
Sprinkler watering yard or water running out of hose

Variations: (1) Have a teammate or friend come up with your list. (2) Exchange lists with a partner. (3) Add more difficult items to the list if you want longer runs. **Bonus Variations:** (1) Use telecommunications to share your scavenger hunt success.

Equipment: One digital camera or cell phone

Sport Scenarios
Objective: To visualize and act out a famous sports scenario in a running manner

Description: Define a running area. Spread out in an area and begin running. Call out a sport scenario and begin running and acting out the scenario. After a designated time period, call out another sports scenario.

Possible sport scenarios to use:
- Winning the Kentucky Derby
- Winning the Indy 500
- Dunking a basketball
- Downhill skiing at the Olympics
- Golf ball hit towards a hole
- Catching a football pass and running towards the end zone for a touchdown
- Swimming at the Olympics
- Outrunning a throw to first
- Riding in the Tour de France
- Outrunning the bulls in the Running of the Bulls

Variations: (1) Come up your own sport scenarios.

Equipment: None needed

Card War

Objective: To sprint to the middle of the playing field and see who has the highest card

Description: Designate a running area with a starting line and end line (recommended 50 to 100 meters long). Place a deck of cards at your end line. Sprint to the end line and draw a card from the top of the pile. Hold your card and jog back to the start line. Lay your 1st card upside down at the starting line. Recover and go again. Continue to sprint to the end line, draw a card and jog back. Continue for a designated number of times.

Keep your stack of picked-up cards in order. Through telecommunications, communicate with a partner who has also performed the Card War game. Compare the first card, then the second card etc. The higher card is the winner, and the winner takes both cards. Keep track of who wins the most number of cards. If there is a tie, keep your card.

Variations: (1) Sprint back instead of jogging back.

Equipment: Playing cards

Run and Pose

Objective: To run and pose for a picture and challenge other runners to run to a spot and take a picture with the same pose

Description: You will need a digital camera or a cell phone camera. During the run, find some photographic locations and pose for pictures. Have fun with this. When the running time period is over, return and share your pictures with other team members via telecommunications.

The challenge will be for each person to do a second run and stop to pose and try to duplicate the poses of everyone else as closely as possible. Place a time period for the run and posing to be accomplished. At the end of the run, everyone comes together online or via text message and shares the photos.

Variations: (1) This doesn't have to take place in a single run. Spread the game out over multiple days, going back and forth with a friend via text message and completing a new pose each run.

Equipment: Digital camera or cell phone with camera

Dice Distance Running

Objective: To break up a distance run into different time periods based upon the roll of dice

Description: Designate a total overall time that you will run. Roll a pair of dice to see how many minutes you will run at one time. When the time is up, return to roll the dice again to determine the next running time.

Dice Distance Running Example				
Overall Running Time Desired: 30-35 minutes				
	Die 1	Die 2	Minutes Run	Cumulative Time
Roll 1	5	4	9	9
Roll 2	2	3	5	14
Roll 3	1	4	5	19
Roll 4	4	6	10	29
Roll 5	2	3	5	34

On the last roll of the dice, if you go over the designated running time, you may stop when you achieve the designated overall time.

Variations: (1) Have someone else roll the dice for you, so that they determine your fate! (2) Vary the length of total running time/number of rolls.

Equipment: Dice

Note: Psychologically, runners may find the overall running time broken down into manageable sections easier than performing a continuous run.

Prediction Runs

Objective: To see how close you can come to your predicted time

Description: Designate a location to run to and back. This is not a race to see how fast you are; the goal is to see how close you can come to your predicted time. You may not look at your watch until you are done with the run. Predict what time you will run for an out and back course. Try to maintain an even pace throughout the run. Keep your pace as you near the finish line. When you cross the line, stop your watch and look at it. Determine how far off your predicted time you were. Record your time to the nearest hundredth of a second. Pick various locations to run to (it is not important to know the distance).

Variations: (1) When done, compare your times to other people and calculate who is best at determining pace. (2) Run several rounds and score as a cross country meet. The closest to the predicted time receives one point, the second closest two points, etc.

Equipment: Stopwatch, recording sheet

Make It-Take It Intervals

Objective: To run intervals and achieve a designated pace time

Description: Determine a pace you want to hit for your interval workout. Run the first interval. If you are within + or − .25 seconds of the assigned interval time (make it), you receive three points. If you are within + or − .5 seconds of the assigned interval time, (make it) you receive two points. If you are within one second + or −, you receive 1 point. If you are not with one second, you will not receive any points. Continue until you have run the desired number of intervals.

Variation: (1) Compare your scores virtually to a teammate. (2) If you are not within a second, you will repeat the interval. (3) Vary the lengths of your intervals.

Equipment: Stopwatch

Scream Team

Objective: To see how far you can run while screaming

Description: Line up on a starting line and start running. As you are running, scream as loud as you can on a single breath. When you can no longer scream, that interval is over. Recover with a jog and then repeat. It's fun to see how far you can go and how loud you can scream! If you get to the edge of a boundary, turn around and come back.

Variations: (1) Note the distance and see if you can go farther next time.

Bonus Variation: (1) Record as video and share with teammates.

Equipment: None needed

Runner's Pentathlon

Objective: To determine what kind of all-around runner you are with a mixture of short and long runs scored decathlon style

Description: You will complete five runs: 1500 meters, 400 meters, 800 meters, 200 meters, 3000 meters, with 10-30 minutes recovery time between runs. Points are scored for each run based on your running time with the use of a decathlon scoring chart. With an equal mix of sprints and distance events, this competition challenges both sprinting and distance abilities to determine how good of an all-around runner you are. Run the 1500 meter. Record your time on the scoring chart. Compare the time to the corresponding points on the scoring tables and record your score in points. Take a recovery (15 minutes for workout, 20-30 minutes if you are using it as a competition). Start the next event the 400 meters and record your time. Record on the scoring chart and record the points off the scoring tables. Keep a running cumulative total. After the last event, calculate your point totals.

Variations: (1) Use a short version of the Runner's Pentathlon by using half of the distances. 800, 200, 400, 100, 1500. In hot weather, the shorter distance is preferred. (2) Compete against others or form a team competition.

Equipment: Scoring chart, scoring tables, stopwatches.

Points	100 meters	200 meters	400 meters	800 meters	1500 meters	3000 meters
1400	9.9	19.78	44.45	1:46.79	3:37.46	7:41.64
1390	9.96	19.9	44.72	1:47.30	3:38.61	7:44.28
1380	10.01	20.02	44.99	1:47.81	3:39.77	7:46.94
1370	10.06	20.14	45.27	1:48.33	3:40.93	7:49.60
1360	10.11	20.26	45.54	1:48.85	3:42.10	7:52.27
1350	10.17	20.38	45.81	1:49.37	3:43.27	7:54.95
1340	10.22	20.5	46.09	1:49.89	3:44.44	7:57.64
1330	10.27	20.62	46.37	1:50.41	3:45.62	8:00.34
1320	10.33	20.74	46.64	1:50.94	3:46.81	8:03.05
1310	10.38	20.86	46.92	1:51.47	3:48.00	8:05.77
1300	10.43	20.99	47.2	1:52.00	3:49.19	8:08.50
1290	10.49	21.11	47.48	1:52.53	3:50.39	8:11.24
1280	10.54	21.23	47.76	1:53.06	3:51.59	8:14.00
1270	10.6	21.36	48.05	1:53.60	3:52.80	8:16.76
1260	10.65	21.48	48.33	1:54.14	3:54.01	8:19.53
1250	10.71	21.61	48.62	1:54.68	3:55.22	8:22.32
1240	10.76	21.73	48.9	1:55.22	3:56.45	8:25.11
1230	10.82	21.86	49.19	1:55.76	3:57.67	8:27.92
1220	10.87	21.99	49.48	1:56.31	3:58.90	8:30.74
1210	10.93	22.12	49.77	1:56.86	4:00.14	8:33.57
1200	10.99	22.24	50.06	1:57.41	4:01.38	8:36.41
1190	11.04	22.37	50.35	1:57.96	4:02.63	8:39.27
1180	11.1	22.5	50.64	1:58.52	4:03.88	8:42.13
1170	11.16	22.63	50.94	1:59.08	4:05.14	8:45.01
1160	11.21	22.76	51.23	1:59.64	4:06.40	8:47.90
1150	11.27	22.89	51.53	2:00.20	4:07.67	8:50.81
1140	11.33	23.02	51.83	2:00.77	4:08.94	8:53.72
1130	11.39	23.15	52.03	2:01.34	4:10.22	8:56.63
1120	11.44	23.29	52.43	2:01.91	4:11.51	8:59.59
1110	11.5	23.42	52.73	2:02.48	4:12.80	9:02.55
1100	11.56	23.55	53.04	2:03.06	4:14.09	9:05.52
1090	11.62	23.69	53.34	2:03.63	4:15.40	9:08.52

1080	11.68	23.82	53.65	2:04.22	4:16.71	9:11.49
1070	11.74	23.96	53.95	2:04.80	4:18.02	9:14.50
1060	11.8	24.09	54.26	2:05.39	4:19.34	9:17.53
1050	11.86	24.23	54.57	2:05.97	4:20.67	9:20.56
1040	11.92	24.37	54.89	2:06.57	4:22.00	9:23.62
1030	11.98	24.5	55.2	2:07.16	4:23.34	9:26.68
1020	12.04	24.64	55.52	2:07.76	4:24.69	9:29.76
1010	12.1	24.78	55.83	2:08.36	4:26.04	9:32.86
1000	12.16	24.92	56.15	2:08.96	4:27.40	9:35.97
990	12.23	25.06	56.47	2:09.57	4:28.77	9:39.10
980	12.29	25.2	56.79	2:10.18	4:30.14	9:42.25
970	12.35	25.35	57.12	2:10.79	4:31.52	9:45.41
960	12.41	25.49	57.44	2:11.41	4:32.91	9:48.58
950	12.48	25.63	57.77	2:12.03	4:34.30	9:51.77
940	12.54	25.78	58.1	2:12.65	4:35.70	9:54.98
930	12.6	25.92	58.43	2:13.28	4:37.11	9:58.21
920	12.67	26.07	58.76	2:13.91	4:38.53	10:01.46
910	12.73	26.22	59.09	2:14.54	4:39.96	10:04.72
900	12.8	26.36	59.43	2:15.17	4:41.39	10:08.00
890	12.86	26.51	59.77	2:15.81	4:42.83	10:11.30
880	12.93	26.66	1:00.10	2:16.64	4:44.28	10:14.61
870	12.99	26.81	1:00.45	2:17.10	4:45.74	10:17.95
860	13.06	26.96	1:00.79	2:17.76	4:47.20	10:21.30
850	13.13	27.11	1:01.13	2:18.41	4:48.68	10:24.68
840	13.19	27.27	1:01.48	2:19.07	4:50.16	10:28.07
830	13.26	27.42	1:01.83	2:19.73	4:51.65	10:31.49
820	13.33	27.57	1:02.18	2:20.40	4:53.15	10:34.92
810	13.4	27.73	1:02.54	2:21.07	4:54.66	10:38.38
800	13.47	27.89	1:02.89	2:21.74	4:56.18	10:41.85
790	13.54	28.04	1:03.25	2:22.42	4:57.71	10:45.35
780	13.61	28.2	1:03.61	2:23.10	4:59.25	10:48.88
770	13.68	28.36	1:03.97	2:23.79	5:00.79	10:52.42
760	13.75	28.52	1:04.34	2:24.48	5:02.35	10:55.99
750	13.82	28.68	1:04.71	2:25.18	5:03.92	10:59.58
740	13.89	28.85	1:05.08	2:25.88	5:05.50	11:03.19
730	13.96	29.01	1:05.45	2:26.59	5:07.09	11:06.83
720	14.03	29.18	1:05.82	2:27.30	5:08.69	11:10.50
710	14.11	29.34	1:06.20	2:28.01	5:10.30	11:14.19
700	14.18	29.51	1:06.58	2:28.73	5:11.93	11:17.90
690	14.25	29.68	1:06.96	2:29.46	5:13.56	11:21.65
680	14.33	29.85	1:07.35	2:30.19	5:15.21	11:25.42
670	14.4	30.02	1:07.74	2:30.93	5:16.87	11:29.21
660	14.48	30.19	1:08.13	2:31.67	5:18.54	11:33.04
650	14.55	30.36	1:08.52	2:32.42	5:20.22	11:36.89
640	14.63	30.54	1:08.92	2:33.17	5:21.92	11:40.78
630	14.71	30.71	1:09.32	2:33.93	5:23.63	11:44.69
620	14.79	30.89	1:09.73	2:34.70	5:25.35	11:48.64
610	14.87	31.07	1:10.13	2:35.47	5:27.09	11:52.62
600	14.94	31.25	1:10.54	2:36.25	5:28.84	11:56.63

590	15.02	31.43	1:10.96	2:37.03	5:30.61	12:00.68
580	15.11	31.62	1:11.37	2:37.82	5:32.29	12:04.76
570	15.19	31.8	1:11.80	2:38.62	5:34.19	12:08.87
560	15.27	31.99	1:12.22	2:39.42	5:36.00	12:13.02
550	15.35	32.18	1:12.65	2:40.24	5:37.83	12:17.21
540	15.43	32.37	1:13.08	2:41.06	5:39.68	12:21.44
530	15.52	32.56	1:13.52	2:41.88	5:41.54	12:25.70
520	15.6	32.75	1:13.96	2:42.72	5:43.43	12:30.01
510	15.69	32.95	1:14.40	2:43.56	5:45.32	12:34.36
500	15.78	33.15	1:14.85	2:44.41	5:47.24	12:38.75
490	15.86	33.35	1:15.31	2:45.27	5:49.18	12:43.18
480	15.95	33.55	1:15.76	2:46.16	5:51.14	12:47.66
470	16.04	33.75	1:16.23	2:47.02	5:53.11	12:52.19
460	16.13	33.96	1:16.70	2:47.91	5:55.11	12:56.77
450	16.22	31.17	1:17.17	2:48.81	5:57.13	13:01.39
440	16.32	34.38	1:17.65	2:49.71	5:59.18	13:06.07
430	16.41	34.59	1:18.13	2:50.63	6:01.24	13:10.80
420	16.51	34.8	1:18.62	2:51.56	6:03.33	13:15.59
410	16.6	35.02	1:19.12	2:52.50	6:05.45	13:20.43
400	16.7	35.24	1:19.62	2:53.45	6:07.59	13:25.33
390	16.8	35.47	1:20.13	2:54.41	6:09.76	13:30.30
380	16.9	35.69	1:20.64	2:55.39	6:11.96	13:35.32
370	17	35.92	1:21.16	2:56.38	6:14.18	13:40.42
360	17.1	36.15	1:21.69	2:57.38	6:16.44	13:45.58
350	17.2	36.39	1:22.23	2:58.39	6:18.73	13:50.82
340	17.31	36.63	1:22.77	2:59.42	6:21.05	13:56.13
330	17.41	36.87	1:23.32	3:00.47	6:23.40	14:01.52
320	17.52	37.12	1:23.88	3:01.53	6:25.79	14:07.00
310	17.63	37.37	1:24.45	3:02.61	6:28.22	14:12.56
300	17.74	37.62	1:25.03	3:03.71	6:30.69	14:18.21
290	17.86	37.88	1:25.62	3:04.82	6:33.20	14:23.95
280	17.97	38.14	1:26.21	3:05.95	6:35.75	14:29.80
270	18.09	38.41	1:26.82	3:07.11	6:38.35	14:35.75
260	18.21	38.68	1:27.44	3:08.28	6:41.00	14:41.81
250	18.33	39.96	1:28.08	3:09.48	6:43.70	14:47.99
240	18.46	39.25	1:28.72	3:10.70	6:46.45	14:54.29
230	18.58	39.53	1:29.38	3:11.95	6:49.27	15:00.73
220	18.71	39.83	1:30.05	3:13.23	6:52.14	15:07.31
210	18.85	40.13	1:30.74	3:14.53	6:55.08	15:14.04
200	18.98	40.44	1:31.45	3:15.87	6:58.09	15:20.93
190	19.12	40.76	1:32.17	3:17.24	7:01.18	15:27.99
180	19.27	41.09	1:32.91	3:18.65	7:04.35	15:35.25
170	19.41	41.42	1:33.67	3:20.10	7:07.60	15:42.71
160	19.57	41.77	1:34.46	3:21.59	7:10.96	15:50.39
150	19.72	42.13	1:35.27	3:23.12	7:14.42	15:58.32
140	19.88	42.49	1:36.11	3:24.71	7:18.00	16:06.51
130	20.05	42.88	1:36.98	3:26.36	7:21.71	16:15.00
120	20.23	43.27	1:37.88	3:28.07	7:25.57	16:23.83
110	20.41	43.69	1:38.82	3:29.86	7:29.59	16:33.03

100	20.6	44.12	1:39.81	3:31.72	7:33.80	16:42.67
90	20.8	44.58	1:40.85	3:33.69	7:38.22	16:52.79
80	21.01	45.06	1:41.94	3:35.77	7:42.90	17:03.50
70	21.24	45.57	1:43.11	3:37.98	7:47.88	17:14.90
60	21.48	46.12	1:44.36	3:40.35	7:52.23	17:27.15
50	21.74	46.72	1:45.72	3:42.94	7:59.04	17:40.46
40	22.03	47.38	1:47.23	3:45.79	8:05.48	17:55.19
30	22.36	48.14	1:48.94	3:49.04	8:12.78	18:11.92
20	22.76	49.03	1:50.97	3:52.88	8:21.45	18:31.75
10	23.27	50.19	1:53.62	3:57.90	8:32.74	18:57.60
0	24.5	53	2:00.00	4:10.00	9:00.00	20:00.00

RELAYS

Run and Get Back
Objective: To perform strides in a relay with a controlled recovery by jogging back to the start of the leg when done

Description:

Traditional Method of Run and Get Back: Normally, you would form a group of four runners to run a 4 x 100 relay. The runners traditionally take a position on the track spread out 100 meters apart from each other. The first runner runs 100 meters and passes the baton (using a visual or non-visual exchange) to the second runner who runs it to the third runner who runs it to the fourth runner who runs it to the finish line. After each individual completes his/her leg, the individual turns around and runs in the opposite direction (clockwise) back to the original starting position. The time aspect of the recovery is controlled because the runners must get back to their original position in time for the next baton exchange. This is a continuous relay that can be continued for a designated time or distance.

Adapted Method: You will have imaginary teammates running with you. After you run 100 meters, imagine and perform the action of handing off to an imaginary runner. Then turn around and jog back to your original starting position. Once you get back to your original start, visualize a teammate coming into hand off to you. Perform receiving an imaginary handoff and continue running. Continue for a designated time or distance.

Variations: (1) Cut across the middle of the infield or your loop to get back to the original starting point to 'take the baton' from the second runner.

Equipment: None

Banana Relay
Objective: To have fun by running with a banana

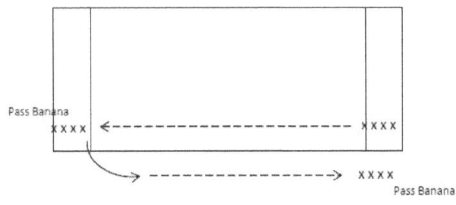

Description: Designate a running area with two end lines. Start at one end line and run to the other. If possible, run barefoot (a soft running surface is preferred for this activity). You will carry a banana as you run. When you get to the far end line, if your shoes are not off, take them off. Lie down on your back. Place the banana between your bare feet and roll over on your back (backwards), extending your legs as far overhead as possible while keeping the banana between your feet. Bring the banana and your feet back to your original starting position. Complete the roll over 10 times, keeping the banana between your feet. This is great for your core. If you drop the banana or touch it with any body part other than your feet, the rep does not count.

After 10 reps (put your shoes back on if you are using them), stand up and sprint back to the starting line. Repeat the routine of doing 10 reps of leg overs with the banana. After all the reps, the banana will be mush! You have the option to peel it and eat it as quickly as possible.

Variations: (1) Leave your shoes on and run to the far end zone. Take off your shoes and socks off and roll over with the banana. Put your shoes back on and run back to the starting line and take your shoes off and rollover with the banana. (2) You may use any other soft, small object. **Bonus Variation:** (1) Take pictures or video and share!

Equipment: One banana or any soft, small object

Wear the Shirt

Objective: To have fun and develop teamwork while changing clothes instead of handing off the baton

Description: Designate a loop course. Have a group of shirts available to put on at starting line. It may be fun to select shirts that have a theme, such as school spirit shirts. Start the first lap with one t-shirt on. Start running on the loop course or track. At the end of the lap, put on a second shirt. Continue the relay by putting on an extra shirt at the conclusion of every lap. How many shirts can you put on?

Bonus Variation: (1) Take some video of your relay run and share it with your teammates. (2) Designate a different theme for each lap.

Equipment: T-shirts

MOTIVATIONAL MOMENTS IN TRACK AND FIELD

Life is often filled with adversity. It is how we adapt and respond to adversity that shapes our successful lives. How can we stay motived to help alleviate the disappointment in life? There are always ways to make ourselves better. Let's focus on what we can control. Be flexible and adapt. Those are traits of successful athletes and people.

One of my favorite quotes is by Jim Rohn. "Don't ask for an easier life, ask for a better you." I encourage you to not waste time feeling sorry for yourself. Spend your time wisely, thinking how you can take adversity and emerge from it as a better person. I have confidence you can do it.

The motivational moments in track and field stories are designed to inspire, encourage, motivate, and teach us valuable life lessons. The stories are written for those who are currently competing, coaching, have participated in track and field, or are simply a track and field or sports fan. The questions at the end of the stories are designed to challenge, teach, and enable you to grow as you apply these principles to athletics and to the bigger game of life.

All of the athletes are ordinary people who used extraordinary desire to accomplish extraordinary things. Each athlete began simply with a dream, which developed into a belief in themselves. They personify the Olympic philosophy – "there are no great people, rather there are great challenges that ordinary people are forced to meet." Their stories offer hope that we can dream and reach beyond our perceived abilities and achieve personal satisfaction.

The stories are rich in history and designed to be read in a few minutes. The stories pay honor to all the young men and women who enter the arena, who make the attempt, and pursue excellence. These stories of great athletes teach us how to eliminate negative thinking, to focus our attention on what is important, and how to overcome obstacles to reach our goals.

Athletes throughout the past century have entered the competitive arena and competed with honor. Although not all athletes are fortunate to catch an Olympic star, all athletes can valiantly reach for the heavens. Their stories of inspiration should be read and remembered. For it has been written, *"The honor should not alone go to those who have not fallen; rather all honor to those who fall and rise again."*

The athletes profiled display the drive, motivation, and dedication to train for years to reach a goal. Their stories teach the values of self-discipline, responsibility, accountability, and loyalty. They demonstrate the qualities necessary to be successful in life—good character, integrity, a strong work ethic, dedication, and perseverance.

You're bound to find motivation and encouragement, no matter what your experience or relationship to track and field. Hopefully you receive pleasure and inspiration from these pages, just as you have found pleasure and inspiration from the greatest sport in the world—track and field.

The most important thing in the Olympic Games is not to win but to take part, just as the most important thing in life is not the triumph but the struggle. The essential thing is not to have conquered but to have fought well. – The Olympic Creed

Roger Bannister: Breaking Through Barriers

Running a 4:00 mile was once deemed impossible. Experts said it was unreachable and dangerous to the health of any athlete who attempted to reach it. Roger Bannister of Great Britain was a 25-year-old medical student at Oxford University completing his internship and putting in long hours at the hospital. His workouts were conducted each day during his 30-minute lunch break. He had been expected to win the 1500 meters at the 1952 Olympics, but Roger was jostled during the race, and never got into contention, finishing fourth.

On May 6, 1954, Roger was scheduled to run at Oxford University's track meet. He had stayed up all night doing his medical rounds and didn't feel like running. But he knew his competitors were closing in on the chase to be the first to run a sub-4:00 mile. He had to go for it! He was paced by a pair of "rabbits," clocking 1:58.2 for the first half-mile. His three-quarter mile time was 3:00.5. With 300 meters to go, Roger said he urged himself "to a supreme effort." He crossed the finish line and began sagging to the ground, drained of all his energy. "It was only then that real pain overtook me," he said. "I felt like an exploded flashlight with no will to live; I just went on existing in the most passive physical state without being unconscious."

The crowd that had urged him on fell silent. Two track officials held him up while spectators converged on him. His time was announced. "Three ... "The rest was drowned out by the cheers. Roger's time of 3:59.4 broke the world record and broke the sub-4:00 barrier, but more importantly, it broke the psychological barrier. What was once deemed impossible had been accomplished. Two years later, 16 runners had logged sub-4:00 miles, accomplishing the one task few thought possible.

Questions for Thought:

1. Roger Bannister's claim to fame was being the first to break the four-minute mile; however, the true significance was breaking through a barrier. What is the significance behind Roger's achievement?

2. Within two years after Roger Bannister broke the 4:00 barrier, 16 people had broken 4:00. Since then, over 1300 people have done so. How can something once thought impossible be achieved by so many people?

3. Think about a barrier that limits you. What can you do to break through the barrier?

Bob Beamon: The Man Who Could Fly

Bob Beamon survived a difficult childhood, as his mother died at age 25 from tuberculosis when Bob was less than a year old. Because his father was in prison, Bob was raised by his grandmother, Bessie. Growing up without a father in a tough neighborhood with violence, gangs, and drugs was challenging, and as a young boy his craving for attention made him a troublemaker in school. Bob struck a teacher, was expelled from school, and sent to an alternative school for delinquents in New York. It was there that Bob realized he could make something of his life and he began to use sports as a means of focusing his attention toward positive goals.

Bob established many school and state records as well as a national record in the triple jump while in high school. Bob attended the University of Texas El Paso (UTEP) and worked on his speed and on a long jumping technique called the hitch kick, where the long jumper runs in the air before landing. He won the NCAA Indoor long jump and triple jump and by age 22, Bob was emerging as one of the top jumpers in the world and was in contention to win an Olympic gold medal in the long jump.

Four months before the Olympic Trials in 1968, Bob was suspended from the UTEP track team and lost his athletic scholarship for participating with other blacks in a boycott of a meet against Brigham Young, a Mormon school whose racial policies disturbed them. The suspension meant that Bob was without a coach. Despite the difficulties he was having at UTEP, Bob won the Olympic Trials long jump, and with the exception of one meet, was undefeated that season. Bob was headed to the 1968 Mexico City Olympic Games as a favorite to win the gold medal, but nobody expected what was about to happen.

Bob accelerated down the long jump runway in the thin air of Mexico City. On each of his 19 strides, he continued to build speed. He hit the board perfectly, exploded off the take-off board to a height of 6-0, ran in the air with his hitch kick, and stretched out his legs to land in the sand pit. Not only was he the first long jumper in history to jump 28-0, he also became the first to reach 29-0, shattering the world record by jumping an unbelievable 29-2½. Of all Olympic records, track and field experts consider none as impressive as the one Bob stunningly set in Mexico City.

Bob Beamon overcame adversity as a child to achieve one of the greatest performances in athletic history at the 1968 Mexico City Olympics. In the world of athletics, a tremendous performance is sometimes referred to as "Beamonesque," a tribute to Bob's outstanding long jump.

Questions for Thought:

1. How did adversity help Bob Beamon achieve success?

2. What limits you in achieving what many may think is impossible?

3. When you get a second chance, how can you make the most of it?

Cliff Cushman: I Dare You!

Cliff Cushman was a remarkably versatile athlete whose talents ranged from a 4:11.6 mile to a sixth place finish in the NCAA triple jump. While attending the University of Kansas, Cliff won the 400-meter hurdles at the 1960 NCAA Championships. He went on to make the U.S. Olympic Team and won a silver medal in the 1960 Olympic Games in Rome in the 400-meter hurdles. He was voted the North Dakota athlete of the year in 1960. Cliff trained hard as he pursued his dream of capturing a gold medal at the 1964 Olympic Games in Tokyo. In the 1964 Olympic Track and Field trials in Los Angeles, Cliff got out strong in the 400-meter hurdles and was on his way to making another Olympic team. However, when he stumbled over a hurdle, he was out of the race and his Olympic dream was over.

After that experience, Cliff wrote a letter to the newspaper in his hometown of Grand Forks, North Dakota, in which he encouraged young people not to feel sorry for him, but instead to set goals for themselves. His letter, written on an airplane only hours after the unfortunate fall, has been an inspiration to many.

After graduating from the University of Kansas in 1961, Cliff became a fighter pilot in the Air Force. In 1966, at the age of 28, as an athlete in the prime of his career, he was listed as missing in action in Vietnam. He left a wife and 10-month-old son. In 1975, Clifton E. Cushman was officially declared dead. But his timeless inspirational message lives on, daring people to become great.

Questions for Thought:

1. Cliff Cushman could have felt sorry for himself after seeing his Olympic gold medal dream shattered when he tripped over a hurdle. How did he respond?

2. What stands out to you in the, "I dare you letter?"

3. What are you willing to "dare to do" in order to become a better athlete?

Raymond Ewry: Legs of Steel

You could say Raymond Ewry had a difficult childhood. He was born in Lafayette, Indiana, and became an orphan at the age of 5. At the age of 7, a doctor told Ray he had polio, which there was no cure for, and he would be bound to a wheelchair, never to walk again. One doctor suggested leg exercises as a last resort. Ray dreamed of getting out of the wheelchair, taking just one step, and being able to walk. Ray would do his exercises several hours a day. He would push himself out of his wheelchair and onto the ground and teach himself to stand. After he could balance himself on his two feet, he began to jump. The crippled boy eventually developed legs of steel.

Ray enrolled at University of Purdue and broke world records in the standing high jump, standing long jump, and standing triple jump. After college, he joined the New York Athletic Club, whose members had taken a strong interest in the inaugural Olympic Games in 1896 in Athens. In 1900, the Olympics were to be held for the second time in Paris, with the New York Athletic Club and Ray competing.

The early Olympic Games consisted of several events such as the standing long, standing triple jump, and standing high jump. These events are no longer contested in current Olympic Games. In the standing high jump, competitors took one step and jumped. Ray jumped 5-5 to win. In the standing long jump, Ray leapt 10-10 to win. In the standing triple jump, Ray covered 34-8½. The French gave Ray the nickname, "The Human Frog."

In the 1904 Olympics in St. Louis, Ray won the same three events again. Two years later, Athens, Greece, was celebrating the 10th anniversary of the modern Games with an extra Olympics competition. Although 1906 was not an Olympic year, the medals counted and Ray won two more. The boy with polio had become the unbeatable Olympic champion. Ray won two more gold medals in London in the 1908 Olympics and retired with 10 gold medals. No other Olympian in history has won as many gold medals without losing a single Olympic competition.

Raymond Ewry, the child who wasn't supposed to take a single step, became one of the greatest jumpers in Olympic history.

Questions for Thought:

1. How has your childhood affected your career?

2. Ray Ewry worked for hours with little progress to show until eventually he developed legs of steel. How long are you willing to work to achieve a goal?

3. Ray was a winner. How would you define being a winner?

Harrison Dillard: Good Things Come to Those Who Wait

Harrison Dillard began hurdling at the age of 8, setting up springs from abandoned car seats as barriers and jumping over them in an alley. In high school, Harrison was very successful, becoming a city and state champion. He attended college at Baldwin Wallace University, but his college years were interrupted when Dillard was called to active duty by the U.S. Army and served two and a half years.

After the war, Harrison went back to Baldwin Wallace to continue his education and was highly successful in track and field, winning numerous titles including National Collegiate Championships in 1946 and 1947 and setting world records in the 120-yard and 220-yard hurdles.

Because of the war, the Olympic Games of 1940 and 1944 were canceled. The revival of the Olympic Games was scheduled for England in 1948. Harrison entered the U.S. 1948 Olympic Trials in the 110-meter hurdles as the Olympic favorite. Harrison almost never hit hurdles when he ran, but that day, he hit the first hurdle and continued to hit hurdles, and suddenly the greatest hurdler in the world was out of the race. His Olympic dream of gold in the hurdles was shattered. Fortunately, he also ran the 100 meters, finishing behind fellow Americans Barney Ewell and Mel Patton, qualifying for the Olympic Games.

A capacity crowd of 75,000 people watched the Olympic Games 100-meter final. Harrison was a big underdog, but got out fast and held the lead the entire way to win Olympic gold. He also came back to add another gold as a member of the 4x100-meter relay team.

Harrison's career was astonishing. He held world records for the 120-yard and 110-meter hurdles, as well as the 220-yard and 200-meter hurdles. His record in the hurdles and sprints was 201 races won and only six lost. But yet, a spark still burned inside of him as he ached over his failure to win an Olympic medal in the hurdles. The 1952 Olympic Games were held in Helsinki, Finland, and Harrison qualified for the Olympic final in the 110-meter hurdles. Harrison led over the third hurdle, but Jack Davis closed fast. Harrison concentrated on maintaining full speed and was careful not to hit a hurdle. At the ninth hurdle, they were even and Harrison relied on his experience to drive over the 10th hurdle and sprint to the finish to win the race.

Harrison Dillard had waited through two Olympiads cancelled because of war, through an Olympiad where he had won gold, but not in his best event, to finally capture the race on which he had set his heart.

Questions for Thought:

1. Harrison had to wait 12 years to finally capture gold in the event he loved. Think of a time when you showed patience and it paid off.

2. How do you motivate yourself to stay committed over a long period of time to reach your goals?

3. Do you have a spark inside you that could lead to success? How do you ignite it?

Rafer Johnson: Role Model

Rafer Johnson was raised in an atmosphere of segregation, discrimination, and poverty in Texas. The Johnson family lived in poverty and at one time even lived in a railroad boxcar for a year. Rafer's athletic career nearly ended before it began when, as a young boy, his left foot was severely cut when it was caught in a conveyor belt.

In high school, Rafer was a superb all-around athlete, winning varsity letters in football, baseball, basketball, and track. In baseball, he hit above .400. In basketball, he averaged 17 points a game, and in football he led the team to three league championships, averaging nine yards a carry as a running back. However, his best sport was track and field.

At UCLA, he turned to the decathlon and in only his fourth decathlon, he broke the world record. He qualified for both the decathlon and the long jump in the 1956 Summer Olympic Games in Melbourne, Australia. However, Rafer suffered an injury before the competition and had to forfeit his place in the long jump. Still suffering from the injury, he finished second behind fellow American Milton Campbell in the decathlon. That would be the last defeat for Rafer in the decathlon.

A car accident one year before the 1960 Rome Olympics left Rafer Johnson with a severely injured back. He spent several weeks in the hospital but recovered enough to win the Olympic Trials. Rafer's biggest challenge in winning the Olympic decathlon was his training partner and fellow UCLA decathlete C.K. Yang of Taiwan. Both trained under legendary UCLA track coach Elvin C. "Ducky" Drake and become close friends. After the first nine events, Johnson led Yang, but Yang was thought to be capable of overcoming this gap in the final event, the 1500 meters. Johnson, however, managed to cling on to Yang in the last event and won the gold. Rafer compiled an Olympic record 8,392 points and earned the title of the greatest all-round athlete in the world. At the age of 25, he had fulfilled his dream of being an Olympic decathlon champion.

Rafer Johnson had the unique ability to overcome both childhood poverty and a severe injury to fulfill his dream of becoming an Olympic champion. He has given his time to serve others, especially in representing the Special Olympics and promoting recreational activities for youth.

Questions for Thought:

1. Rafer overcame a challenging period as a youth to turn into an exemplary role model. Who are you a role model to?

2. Knowing that you are a role model to someone, how does that affect your actions?

3. Rafer's teammate, C.K. Yang, challenged him in practice every day and challenged him to win the gold medal. How does having other talented people around every day help you?

Eric Liddell: Pure Gold

Eric Liddell was born in China in 1902 to Scottish missionaries. He went to school in China until the age of 5, when he was enrolled in a boarding school in England. Eric participated in cricket and made the Scottish national rugby team as a youth before his natural running ability began to emerge.

The 1924 Olympics were in Paris, France. Eric had become one of the top sprinters in the world and was the favorite to win the 100 meters. When the Olympics' schedule was published months before the games, a 100-meter heat was scheduled for a Sunday. However, Eric was a devout Christian and refused to run in a heat held on the Sabbath. A man of strong principles, Eric withdrew from his best event, the 100 meters. Eric had limited previous success in the 400 meters, but since the 400-meter was not being held on a Sunday, he could participate in that event. He had also been selected to run as a member of the 4x100-meter and 4x400-meter relay teams at the Olympics but declined to run those as their heats were to be run on a Sunday as well.

Eric first competed in the 200 meters and won the bronze medal in Paris. He went to the starting line of the 400-meter race as a big underdog. Before 1928, the 400 meters was considered a middle distance event in which runners raced the first curve and coasted through the backstretch. Eric ran hard the entire first 200 meters to get ahead of the favored Americans. The Americans challenged him all the way down the home straight, but Eric held on to take the win, breaking the Olympic record with a time of 47.6.

At the peak of his athletic career, Eric left Scotland to devote his life to being a missionary in China. Eric chose to live a dangerous life in China, serving his God. His greatness of heart and unwavering conviction are an inspiration to people of faith everywhere. In 1941, life in China had become dangerous because of Japanese aggressiveness. Despite suffering many hardships, Eric refused to leave. The Japanese imprisoned Eric, and suffering from overwork and malnourishment, he died of a brain tumor in a prison camp a few months before the end of World War II. Eric's story was portrayed in the popular movie, Chariots of Fire. Eric Liddell upheld the Olympic motto, "Citius, Altius, Fortius" which means, "Swifter, Higher, Stronger," throughout his life.

Questions for Thought:

1. Eric's beliefs were so strong that he was willing to give up Olympic glory. On a scale of 1-10 (10 high), how strong are your beliefs?

2. There is a saying, "if you don't stand for something, you will fall for anything." What do you stand for?

3. Eric had a passion to help people and gave his life for it. What sacrifices have you made to help people?

Joe Kovacs: Throwing Out of the Parking Lot Ring

On the road to Rio, Joe Kovacs encountered much heartbreak. At a young age, Joe lost his father to colon cancer. Just hours later, his grandmother passed away of heart failure. "It was sad losing my father and him not being there, but my mom stepped up so much and provided so much for me," he says. "It was never, 'look down upon yourself,' it was always 'keep looking forward.'

Joe began throwing in a parking lot in high school, with his mom as his coach. He didn't have a track or a throwing circle, so they went out to the parking lot, and started drawing chalk lines. He eventually became good enough to earn a scholarship to Penn State University.

At the 2012 U.S. Olympic Trials, in his last meet wearing a Penn State jersey, Kovacs stood in third place in the standings, the final qualifying position for the London Games, after his third of six throws. However, 2009 World champion Christian Cantwell jumped ahead of Kovacs, who would finish in fourth place, one spot shy of becoming the youngest American to make the Olympics in the event in 20 years. Still, Kovacs had thrown a personal best at the biggest meet of his life, coming in with no expectations of cracking the top three.

Joe represented Team USA in the 2015 World Championships and won a gold medal with a record throw of 71-11 ½. Kovacs trained at the U.S. Olympic Training Center at Chula Vista with Olympic teammates Ryan Crouser and Darrell Hill. His training included gymnastic movements such as high bar swings and front and back handsprings.

Kovacs took 2nd at the 2016 Olympic Trials shot put, throwing 72-0 ¼ behind Ryan Crouser's lifetime best of 72-6 ½.

Joe took the early lead in the Olympic final throwing 71-5 ½, which would prove to be his best throw and good enough to capture the silver medal after teammate Crouser's Olympic record.

Questions for Thought:

1. Joe suffered family tragedy with the loss of loved ones but continued to look forward. How do you see past your problems to the future?

2. Joe's mom adapted by creating a ring out of a parking lot. Think of a story where you overcame the odds.

3. Joe finished only one spot out of the Olympic team in 2012 and worked harder to make the team in 2016. What are some things you have learned from failing?

Aries Merritt: Transplant to Success

Aries Merritt was on top of the world in 2012, with an Olympic gold medal and a world record of 12.80 seconds in the 110-meter hurdles, and he recorded the most sub-13-second races in a single season by any athlete. In 2015, Aries Merritt was on top of an operating table.

His kidneys began to fail in 2013 and he was told he might never run again as a result of collapsing focal segmental glomerulosclerosis, a progressive form of kidney disease. The diagnosis turned Aries into a depressed, angry, and mean person. He battled this illness with kidneys functioning at only 10 percent to win a bronze medal at the 2015 world championships in a season-best time, just a week before undergoing his kidney transplant thanks in part to his sister, who served as his kidney donor.

Doctors told Aries he had to wait eight weeks to return to training. He was able to get going in seven, then needed to wait several more weeks when his new kidney needed a second surgery in October. After a single day of training, he had developed a hematoma. Aries didn't lift weights for two months after surgery. He takes medication for his kidney every 12 hours, but the drugs are either neutral or could slightly weaken muscles.

Though maybe not as strong, Aries felt as though he was in better shape than ever going into the 2016 Olympic Trials. Approximately 10 months post-surgery, he had also been recovering from a torn groin in recent weeks. Aries launched from the starting blocks in the 110-meter hurdles final, his trail leg grazing the transplant scar across his abdomen 10 times as he cleared each hurdle. An agonizing wait for the time to show up on the scoreboard showed that Aries missed the 2016 Olympic team by the cruelest of margins: one one-hundredth of one second. Aries thought he finished second or third and asked for the photo finish to be review, but the result stood.

Despite barely missing his second Olympic team, Aries Merritt still holds the world record in the 110-meter hurdles. But more importantly, he has set the standard for courageous effort.

Questions for Thought:
1. With his kidneys only operating at 10%, Aries won a silver medal in the 2015 World Championships. What is your reaction to this performance?

2. Aries couldn't wait to resume training. How anxious are you to improve your game?

3. What does courage mean to you?

Edwin Moses: An Enduring Streak

Edwin Moses' high school basketball coach cut him from the team and the football coach kicked him off the team for fighting. He took up track and started running the hurdles and 440-yard dash. Rather than accept an athletic scholarship to a more powerful track and field program, Edwin accepted an academic scholarship in physics and engineering to Morehouse College in Atlanta, Georgia.

Edwin had run only one 400-meter hurdle race prior to running the 400-meter hurdles in March of 1976. It was only five months away from the Olympic Games in Montreal. Despite being a novice at the event, he advanced quickly. Every world class hurdler was taking 14 steps between the hurdles; however, Edwin started taking an unprecedented 13 steps between hurdles. At the Olympic Trials, Edwin won the 400-meter hurdles and set an American record with a time of 48.30.

Edwin was competing in his first international meet at the Montreal Olympics, where he won the gold, setting a world record of 47.64. His eight meter victory over U.S. teammate Mike Shine was the largest winning margin ever in that event in the Olympics. He had accomplished the extraordinary feat of becoming the 400-meter hurdles Olympic champion and world record holder in his first year of running the event. For the next decade, he dominated the 400-meter hurdles with the longest winning streak achieved by an individual athlete in track and field. Edwin was unbeatable on the track, but politics prevented him from winning his second Olympic gold when President Carter ordered the United States Olympic teams to boycott the 1980 Olympics.

At the 1984 Olympics in Los Angeles, Edwin became only the second man to win the Olympic 400- meter hurdles twice. One of the greatest honors and most memorable moments of his career came when he was chosen to recite the Athletes' Oath during the opening ceremonies in Los Angeles. He came back four years later at the 1988 Olympic Games in Seoul to finish third in the final race of his career.

Edwin was the dominant 400-meter hurdler in track and field for more than a decade. His 107 straight wins in a period of almost 10 years is the longest winning streak ever in track and field, and is considered one of the top winning streaks in all of sports. He was a strong advocate against steroid use and performance enhancing drugs. His phenomenal rise to world prominence by becoming an Olympic champion in his first year running an event was a remarkable achievement.

Questions for Thought:

1. Edwin Moses did not use being a novice as an excuse, as he won an Olympic medal only five months after first running the 400-meter hurdles. When you first begin a task, what do you focus on?

2. What are some keys to consistently performing well over a long period of time?

3. Edwin took a strong stand against the use of performance enhancing drugs. How strong is your stand against performance enhancing drugs?

Dan O'Brien: World's Greatest Athlete

Dan O'Brien was born in Portland, Oregon, where his parents gave him up for adoption at birth. Dan was talented but lacked commitment to develop his skills. Eventually, Dan made the commitment to be the "best athlete in the world" and turned to the decathlon. Coached by Mike Keller and Rick Sloan, Dan improved to become a top decathlete.

Dan set the world record in the decathlon and was favored to win the Olympic gold medal in 1992. Reebok created a popular TV advertising campaign featuring U.S. rivals Dave Johnson and Dan.

The commercials, entitled "Dan & Dave," were meant to build interest in Reebok and the decathletes, culminating in the 1992 Summer Olympics in Barcelona. However, at the 1992 U.S. Olympic Trials in New Orleans, Dan, seeking to conserve his energy in the hot and humid conditions, passed on the lower heights in the pole vault. When he entered the competition at 15-9, he failed in his first two attempts at his opening height. Dan was down to one more jump. Unfortunately, he missed on his third and final attempt, resulting in no points for the event and he did not qualify for the Olympic team. His unexpected failure caused Reebok to revise new ads featuring Dan cheering on Dave, who went on to win the bronze medal.

Dan went to work the next four years to prepare for the 1996 Olympic Games in Atlanta. Dan won all eight decathlons he entered, won two world championships by impressive margins, and set a world record of 8,891 points. For Dan to win the 1996 Olympics, he had to qualify for the U.S. team. This was a challenge he had failed at in the last Olympic Trials. The ghosts of failure were on his mind as he stood on the pole vault runway at the 1996 Olympic Trials in Atlanta. With his 15-foot fiberglass pole, he ran down the runway, planted his pole, and soared over the bar. His failure at the 1992 Trials was behind him.

Under intense pressure of competing in his home country as the world record holder, he rose to the challenge, earning the title as "the world's greatest athlete" as he captured the decathlon gold at the 1996 Summer Olympics in Atlanta, Georgia.

Questions for Thought:

1. Dan failed to make the team in 1992 and had nightmares about the miss. Eventually, he put it out of his mind to be successful. How do you forget about past mistakes?

2. It took Dan a while before he eventually made a commitment to use his talent. How can you make a commitment to use the talent you have?

3. How can a failure motivate you?

Al Oerter: Competitor

The word that best describes Al Oerter is "competitor." He is the only athlete to win four gold medals at four successive Olympiads and set four consecutive Olympic records. At Sewanhaka High School in New York, he was a sprinter and then a miler. As he was running at practice one day, a discus landed near his feet. He picked it up and casually threw it back. His coach noticed that he threw it back farther than the discus throwers were throwing it. So, Al became a discus thrower. He set the national high school record, and then attended the University of Kansas, where he won two NCAA titles. While at Kansas, Al competed in his first Olympics at the 1956 Summer Games in Melbourne. He was not considered the favorite but won gold after he unleashed a throw of 184-11, which was a personal best and Olympic record.

An automobile accident at the age of 20 nearly killed him, but he recovered in time to compete at the 1960 Summer Olympics in Rome. Al threw the discus 194-2, setting an Olympic record and winning his second gold medal. During the early 1960s, Al continued to have success, setting his first world record in 1962 as he became the first man to throw more than 200 feet in the discus. He was considered a heavy favorite to win a third gold medal in Tokyo in 1964. However, he was bothered by a neck injury, and six days before the competition, he slipped on a wet concrete discus circle and tore rib cartilage on his throwing side, causing internal bleeding and severe pain. Team doctors told him not to throw for six weeks. He refused. "These are the Olympics," he was quoted as saying at the time. "You die before you quit." Competing in great pain, Al set a new Olympic record and won a third Olympic gold medal.

Al returned to the Olympics in 1968 at Mexico City. However, experts felt that at age 32, he was too old to win. Rising to the occasion, as he always did in the Olympic Games, Al released another personal record and another Olympic record throw of 212-6 to win and become the first track and field athlete to win four consecutive gold medals. Al Oerter retired from athletics after the 1968 Olympics. He did make an attempt to qualify for the American team in 1980 at the age of 43, but he finished fourth, one spot from making the Olympic team. However, he did set his overall personal record of 227-10¾ that year.

Questions for Thought:

1. Al Oerter rose to the occasion to set a personal record in every Olympic Games he competed in. What is the key to rising to the occasion?

2. Al threw in severe pain instead of quitting. On a scale of 1-10, (10 high) what is your pain tolerance?

3. At the age of 43, Al achieved a new personal record. How do you maintain that high of a performance level for that long?

Steve Prefontaine: A Work of Art

During his brief 24-year life, Steve Prefontaine grew from hometown hero, to record-setting college phenomenon, to internationally acclaimed track star. Since his death in 1975, Pre has become a legend. He combined talent, discipline (he never missed a workout in four years of college), and determination with a personality that gained him many fans who came to watch him run, roaring with cheers of "Go Pre!"

Pre developed his hunger to be the best at Marshfield High School in Coos Bay, Oregon. As a freshman at Marshfield High School, he placed 53rd in the state cross country meet. Prefontaine ran a personal best time of 5:01 in the mile his freshman year. Determined to improve, Pre undertook a high mileage training plan during the summer and the following year, he placed sixth in the state cross country meet. However, in his sophomore track and field season, he failed to qualify for state. Motivated, he continued to train hard and his junior and senior years proved highly successful. He won every meet, including the state meet, and set a national high school record his senior year in the two-mile race with a time of 8:41.5.

Pre ran for the University of Oregon and won three NCAA Cross Country Championships and four straight three-mile titles in track and field. Following his freshman year, he went undefeated. He was known for going out hard and not relinquishing the lead, a tactic that his fans and fellow competitors admired.

He set the American record at 5000 meters during the 1972 Olympic Games in Munich. Pre led nearly the entire last mile in a fierce battle with Lasse Viren of Finland but was passed with 150 meters to go and finished fourth.

Before his tragic death in a car accident in 1975, Prefontaine held every American record from the 2,000 meters to the 10,000 meters. He is considered one of the greatest American runners of all time.

Questions for Thought:

1. What made Pre such a great runner?

2. Years after his death, Pre is still considered a legend. Why?

3. What do you think is the most admirable quality Pre possessed?

Derek Redmond: Determined to Finish

Derek Redmond, of Great Britain, arrived at the 1992 Summer Olympic Games in Barcelona determined to win a medal. Although he did not achieve his goal, his performance over 400 meters became one of the most inspiring performances in Olympic history.

Derek first started a successful track career in Great Britain at the age of 7. It didn't take him long to become the British champion and record holder at 400 meters. He set the British record for the 400-meter run at the age of 19 when he ran 44.82, which he later improved to 44.50. However, injuries consistently plagued Derek's career. He had 13 operations on his Achilles tendons and knees and it forced him to pull out of many major competitions. In the 1988 Games in Seoul, South Korea, he was forced to withdraw just 10 minutes before the race because of an Achilles injury.

The 1992 Olympics were Derek's stage and it was his time to shine and show the world his remarkable talent. Derek came into the Barcelona Games as the British record holder and in the best shape of his life. In the first round, he ran the fastest time of all the runners in the field. In the semifinal, his dad, Jim, sat in the stands supporting Derek as he did at all his competitions. As the gun sounded for the race, Derek started well and quickly took the lead. In the backstretch at the 200-meter mark, he appeared to be a lock to make the finals. Suddenly, he heard a loud pop in his right hamstring, as if he had been shot. His momentum kept him hobbling until he fell to the ground in pain. Painfully, he arose and with his leg quivering, he began to hop on one leg before falling to the track. Medical personnel ran to assist him.

Derek's Olympic dream of winning a medal was once again gone. With tears streaming down his face, Derek waved off the stretcher offered by the medical crew. He struggled to get to his feet and started hobbling down the track, the pain and agony etched deeply in his face. Derek was going to finish, not for the crowd, but for himself. One painful step at a time, Redmond limped toward the finish line. Derek's father raced down from the top of the stands to help his son, dodging security who tried to stop him.

When Jim reached his son, Derek put an arm around his father for support and the two of them slowly made their way around the track to the finish line. The full stadium of 65,000 spectators, cheering, clapping, and crying, rose to give the Redmonds a standing ovation. Derek's determination to finish the race has become one of the most inspiring races in Olympic history.

Questions for Thought:

1. Have you ever almost quit something because it was hard, but with determination, you carried on?

2. How does it feel when you reach an accomplishment that you almost gave up on?

3. Derek Redmond's father was there to help him finish. Who is on your support staff? How do they help you reach your goals?

Louis Zamperini: Devil at His Heels

Louis Zamperini was a juvenile troublemaker that had a knack for getting into trouble, so his brother got him to go out for high school track. Louie ran the mile in 4:21.2 and set a new national high school record. He went to the University of Southern California and competed in the U.S. Olympic Trials in 1936. Louie finished second in the 5000 meters at the trials to qualify for the Olympics to be held in Berlin, Germany. He finished eighth in the Olympic 5000-meter final, running the last lap in a blazing 56 seconds, catching the attention of Adolf Hitler. Upon returning to college in 1938, Louie set a national collegiate mile record, which stood for 15 years. He was also a part of many national record-breaking relay teams. He may have broken the four-minute mile had he not joined the United States Army Air Force as a bombardier in the South Pacific during World War II.

Louie was deployed to Hawaii, and after flying a number of missions his aircraft was shot down. Louie and two other soldiers lived through the crash in the Pacific Ocean. The soldiers had hope that search planes would rescue them. Fighting storms, sharks, lack of drinking water and food, as well as enemy attacks, the soldiers drifted day after day on a small raft. After 47 days adrift in the ocean, the Japanese Navy rescued Louie and the only other surviving soldier. The Japanese held Louie in captivity in a brutal prisoner camp. One particular guard wanted to make an example of the eternally optimistic Olympic runner, and for two years the guard tried to break Louie's spirit with verbal and physical cruelty. He faced daily beatings, inhumane treatment, and lack of food. His weight dropped from 160 pounds before the plane crash to 67 pounds. The threat of mass execution was constant for two and a half years until the end of the war. He was listed as killed in action and his family feared he was dead. Despite all the difficulties, Louie focused on keeping his mind sharp and maintaining a positive spirit.

After the war was over, Louie returned to a hero's welcome but that did not last long. He had hopes of coming back to run in the Olympics again, but war injuries would not allow him to train. He constantly had bad nightmares and turned to alcohol.

His life changed when he met evangelist Billy Graham, who helped him launch a new career as a Christian inspirational speaker. One of his favorite themes was "forgiveness," and he visited many of the guards from his prison camp days to let them know that he had forgiven them.

Questions for Thought:

1. Louis Zamperini spent 47 days on a raft without food and water but kept up his positive attitude. What can you learn from this story?

2. Often times, we think we have it tough. Does Louie's story make you believe you have it easy? How could you toughen up?

3. Louie forgave the guards that committed some of the worst war crimes in history. How do you rate your ability to forgive on a scale of 1-10 (10 high)?

Gretel Bergmann: Betrayed

Gretel Bergmann was the daughter of a wealthy Jewish entrepreneur who quickly discovered her passion for athletics. She excelled to become Germany's national female high jump champion during the 1930s. But shortly after Adolf Hitler seized power in 1933, the harassment began. Jews were ostracized and unfairly discriminated against. Despite previously being named a member of the German Olympic team, she was no longer welcome to train at her club or with her longtime coach and was denied the opportunity to compete.

When Gretel was 19 years old, she was sent by her parents to live in England with a goal of competing for Great Britain in the 1936 Olympic Games. After winning the 1934 British high jump championship, the Nazis ordered her to return to Germany in 1936. The United States had threatened to boycott the Olympic Games because of the persecution of Jews in Germany, and the Nazi propaganda machine needed to present a token Jew at the games. Facing threats to her family if she did not return home and compete for Germany, Gretel returned.

The training conditions back in Germany were horrible. However, Gretel overcame the adversity and tied the German and European high jump record of 5-3. Two weeks later, German sport authorities delivered a letter stating that her achievement was not good enough to represent Germany in the Olympics. Being denied the opportunity was what she described as "the worst moment of my life," because Gretel relished the opportunity to show that a Jewish girl could be as good as anybody else.

Ironically, at the same time, the United States was setting sail for the Berlin Games. The controversial Olympic boycott movement had failed, with top U.S. officials convinced that there was not mistreatment of the Jews in Germany. The gold medal in the high jump went to Hungarian Ibolya Csak who was, ironically, Jewish. The bronze went to the German "Aryan" Elfriede Kaun. A year after the 1936 Olympic Games, Gretel immigrated to the United States and won the U.S. women's high jump and shot put championships in 1937 and the high jump title again in 1938. Gretel would eventually became a U.S. citizen. When World War II began and the Olympics scheduled to be held in 1940 and 1944 were cancelled, Gretel's Olympic dream was over. Gretel Bergmann's Olympic story is one of triumph and betrayal. Gretel was denied the opportunity to prove she was among the best.

Questions for Thought:

1. Gretel faced tremendous discrimination in her attempts to compete as an athlete. What is the greatest difficulty you have faced? How did you overcome the difficulty?

2. Athletics is a privilege to be able to participate in. How much do you appreciate the privilege to have that opportunity?

3. Gretel had no facilities to train in yet improvised and set records. What are some ways you have improvised and have successfully overcome barriers?

Joan Benoit Samuelson: No Guts, No Glory

Joan Benoit Samuelson is one of the all-time greatest marathoners the world has ever seen. Her dedication and courageous running took her to the top of the running world, making history in the process. Joan took to long distance running to help recover from a broken leg suffered while skiing.

At Bowdoin College, she excelled in athletics for two years and then transferred to North Carolina State to focus on running, earning All-America honors. She entered the 1979 Boston Marathon as a relative unknown. She won the race in 2:35:15, taking eight minutes off the course record. She repeated that success with a record-setting victory again in 1983, taking more than two minutes off the world's best time.

In the months leading up to the 1984 U.S. Olympic Marathon Trials, Joan was hampered by a knee injury. With just 17 days to go before the Olympic Trials race, Joan visited an orthopedic surgeon, who advised her to have an arthroscopic procedure to release the plica, a small band of tissue that was causing her knee to lock. Joan took his advice, had the surgery and the day after surgery immediately got back into training, working out on a hand ergometer (moving pedals with your hands and arms). Amazingly, just 17 days later, Joan made the U.S. Olympic marathon team.

History was made at the 1984 Olympic Games hosted by Los Angeles. It was the first ever women's Olympic Marathon. Women had come a long way since 1928, when it was deemed too exhaustive for women to run over 200 meters in a race. The field included marathon legends Grete Waitz, Rosa Mota, and Ingrid Kristianson. Few of the Olympic runners knew who Joan was, so when she went to the lead early, they didn't worry about her and hung back. In the hot and smoggy conditions, the small runner with a big heart and desire continued to pound out mile after mile and won the first Olympic women's marathon in a time of 2:24:52, more than a minute ahead of her rivals.

Joan has continued to be a role model for women's running. She has written books and is a motivational speaker and a coach. She still runs competitively and for fun. At the age of 50 she ran the 2008 U.S. Olympic Marathon Trials in 2:48:08, making her the only woman to run sub-2:50 marathons over five decades.

A pioneer in women's distance running, Joan qualified for seven Olympic Marathon Trials. She is an inspiration to women and runners throughout the world that with dreams and dedication, challenging goals can be achieved.

Questions for Thought:

1. How did Joan handle her injuries?

2. Although not the race favorite, how did Joan approach the Olympic Marathon in 1984?

3. How can you run with guts to achieve the glory?

Fanny Blankers-Koen: The Flying Housewife

Francina "Fanny" Blankers-Koen, a Dutch athlete, competed during a time when the sports public disregarded women's athletics. She started track and field at the age of 17, and in only her third race, she set a national record in the 800 meters. However, the 800 meters was considered too physically demanding for female contestants and had been removed from the Olympic program after 1928. So Fanny, at 18 years of age, made the Dutch team as a sprinter and high jumper. At the 1936 Berlin Olympics, she placed fifth in the high jump and ran a leg on the fifth place 4x100-meter relay team.

Her opportunity to compete in another Olympics was denied by the cancellation of the 1940 and 1944 Olympics due to World War II. Fanny managed to set world records in the sprints, hurdles, high jump, and long jump during the war years. However, training was not easy due to the war. Sport was the last thing on peoples' minds.

When Fanny gave birth to her first child, it was automatically assumed her career would be over, as top female athletes who were married were rare at the time, and it was considered inconceivable that a mother could be an athlete. Fanny had other plans though, and she resumed training just weeks after her son's birth, earning the nickname "The Flying Housewife." Although she held six world records at the time, many believed that a 30-year-old mother of two was too old to be an athlete and should stay home.

At the 1948 Olympics in London, her first win was the 100 meters, and she became the first Dutch athlete to win an Olympic title in track and field. She won a second gold in a tight 80-meter hurdle finish. Fanny picked up a third gold in the 200-meter dash, which was the first time the women's 200 meters had been held. In her fourth and final event, the 4x100-meter relay, Fanny was running the anchor when she received the baton in third place, some five meters behind Australia and Canada. Burning the straightaway, she passed both runners ahead of her to win gold for her country.

At age 34, she took part in her third Olympics at the 1952 Helsinki Games, but she hit a hurdle, which took her out of the race. It was her last major competition. Fanny Blankers-Koen's last moment of glory came in 1999, when the International Association of Athletics Federations (I.A.A.F.) declared her the "Female Athlete of the Century."

Questions for Thought:

1. It was once thought that most of the track and field events were too strenuous for women to compete in. How has history proven that wrong?

2. During Fanny's time, 30-years-old was deemed too old, and being a mother and an athlete was considered inconceivable. What has changed since the 1940s?

3. Although she missed two Olympics canceled due to war, Fanny was named "Female Athlete of the Century." What would it be like to miss the prime of your career?

Michelle Carter: Shot Put Diva

Michelle Carter didn't even know her father, Michael Carter, had won an Olympic medal and a Super Bowl ring in the same year. That is, until a junior high teacher encouraged her to try the shot put.
Her father ensured the shot put had been her choice and had been careful not to put any pressure on Michelle to follow in his footsteps, as he had won silver in the shot put in the 1984 Olympics. But as it turns out, she did.

Her career began by earning a silver medal at the 2001 World Youth Championships, the first time she had gone out of the country to throw. Since then, she has become a force to reckon with on the international scene. She competed in the 2008 Beijing Olympics, where she finished just 15th. Since 2012, though, she has finished in the top five at all six major global championships indoor and outdoor and finished 5th at the London Olympics.

But after the 2012 Olympics, she became tired, frustrated, and developed low self-esteem when her off-season weight gain didn't come off when she returned to her training regimen and was ultimately diagnosed with hypothyroidism.

Although ninety pounds heavier, Michelle didn't allow her condition to affect the person she was inside. She is a proponent of positive body image and runs a positive sports confidence camp for young female throwers. Considering herself to be a girly-girl, Michelle, a certified professional make-up artist, has been deemed the "Shot Put Diva." She also posed for ESPN's body issue and tries to encourage and send young women the message that muscles are cool.

These are the very same muscles that helped propel Michelle to an American Record in 2013, throwing 66-4 ¾, a throw that would send her confidence into a whirlwind, gaining momentum with each competition. In Rio, it appeared New Zealand's Valerie Adams would win her third consecutive gold medal in the event when Carter stepped into the ring for her final throw. She had come from behind to win her last two major championships, the 2016 World Indoors (where she set an American Indoor record) and the Olympic Trials on her final throw. Michelle Carter catapulted the shot 67-8 ¼, breaking the American Record and becoming the first American woman to capture gold in the event.

Questions for Thought:

1. Michelle's father was an Olympic silver medalist but did not push Michelle into the sport. How do you handle expectations?

2. Michelle has struggled with thyroid problems but is a role model encouraging others on self-esteem. Is your self-esteem separate from your athletic performance?

3. Michelle has learned to adapt and thrive in big moments. How can your routine develop the confidence for you to perform when it counts?

Alice Coachman: African American Pioneer

Alice Coachman became the first black woman of any nationality to win a gold medal at the Olympics with her victory in the high jump at the 1948 Summer Games in London. Alice was born as the middle child to a family of 10 children in rural Georgia. Because her parents were poor, Alice had to pick cotton to help her family meet expenses while she was in elementary school. She liked to run, but her father would whip her when he caught her running because, "women weren't supposed to be running like that." But secretly, Alice continued to practice. Unable to afford shoes, she ran barefoot on the dirt roads near her house, practicing jumps over a crossbar made of rags tied together. Eventually, her parents, although still reluctant, allowed her to compete in track and field to improve her raw talent. She broke high school and then collegiate records by the time she was 16 years old.

Alice's biggest goal was to compete in the Olympic Games in 1940. But World War II forced the cancellation of the 1940 and 1944 Olympic Games. Alice became the U.S. national high jump champion and the first African American women selected for a U.S. Olympic team. On August 7, 1948, at age 25, Alice made history by becoming the first woman of African descent to win an Olympic gold medal. The high jump competition came down to D.J. Tyler of England and Alice, with both jumping an Olympic record 5-6 1/4; however, Alice won with the least number of misses.

Alice became the first African American woman to endorse an international product when the Coca-Cola Company featured her prominently on billboards along America's highways. Alice Coachman's Olympic gold medal paved the way for generations of African American athletes to achieve great success.

Questions for Thought:

1. Alice ran barefoot and practiced with a cross bar made of rags. How are some ways you have improvised to get the job done?

2. Do you feel it is a privilege or a right to participate in sports?

3. Women were not supposed to be running during Alice's era. What would you do if the right to participate in athletics was taken away from you?

Gail Devers: Recovering to Achieve

Gail Devers was a shining young talent in the 100 meters and 100-meter hurdles. Her training program was going well for the 1988 Olympic Games, when she started suffering from headaches and vision loss. She was able to qualify for the U.S.A Olympic team in the 100-meter hurdles but was eliminated in the semifinals. After the Olympics, Gail's health continued to decline further.

Doctor after doctor failed to diagnose her illness, as she suffered debilitating fatigue, losing nearly all her hair. After more than two years, Gail was finally diagnosed with a thyroid disease. She was treated with radioactive iodine to disable her thyroid. Fearing she would be banned from competition for using banned substances, Gail refused the drugs that were intended to diminish side effects from the radiation therapy required to treat her enlarged thyroid. Gail developed excruciatingly painful lesions on her feet and sores and scales all over her body and face. Her weight dropped from 125 to only 87 pounds, as she grew weaker and weaker. Gail was so distraught over her appearance that she covered all the mirrors in her Los Angeles home.

Her feet swelled so severely that the 5-3 runner could squeeze only into a size-12 men's sneaker and eventually she couldn't walk at all. Family members had to carry her to the bathroom. Her feet grew so swollen and infected that medical authorities believed they might require amputation, a diagnosis Gail fought against. Eventually, recovery came as Gail began a lifelong program of thyroid hormone replacement therapy.

Remarkably, Gail began to run again. At first, she rode a stationary bike at trackside, then she walked, then jogged, and eventually began to sprint and jump. The amazing Gail not only ran, she qualified for the 1992 Olympics Games in both the 100-meter hurdles and 100-meter dash. The Barcelona Olympics 100-meter dash was one of the closest in history, with five women within six one-hundredths of a second. After a long wait for results, the photo finish showed Gail as the winner. In the finals of the hurdles, she was leading into the final hurdle when disaster struck as she hit the last hurdle, stumbling across in fifth place.

In 1996, Gail again qualified for both the 100 meters and 100-meter hurdles Olympic final in Atlanta. In the 100-meter final, Merlene Ottey of Jamaica and Gail finished in the same time, with neither knowing who had won. Both were awarded the same time, but Gail was judged to have finished first. In the final of her favorite event, the 100-meter hurdles, she finished fourth.

Questions for Thought:

1. Gail Devers, recognized for competing with her long nails and powerful speed, left a legacy of a lesson about recovery and achievement. What did you learn from the story?

2. How do your problems compare to what Gail went through?

3. How do you stay determined when facing adversity?

Lolo Jones: Backbone of Steel

Lori (Lolo) Jones has overcome many hurdles in her life to excel in track and field. Lolo was raised by a single mother with five children while her father spent most of her childhood in prison. Her family was poor and had to move often, once even living in a church basement. As she entered high school, she parted ways with her mother and stayed with four different families throughout her time in high school. Her high school career drew the attention of Louisiana State University, where Lolo developed into one of the best collegiate hurdlers in the country, becoming a multi-time NCAA champion.

In 2004, Lolo ran in the Olympic Trials but failed to make the Olympic team. As she contemplated her future, she knew she would have to make sacrifices and work several part-time jobs in order to make it work financially. But her heart was still in track and field.

She entered the 2008 Olympic Games as a favorite and opened a slight lead in the finals of the 100- meter hurdles. With only two hurdles remaining, Lolo was just a few meters from Olympic gold. She was just a couple of seconds from accomplishing her lifetime dream. However, tragedy struck on the next to last hurdle as she tripped and stumbled, dropping to seventh place.

She would have to wait four more years for another opportunity. The pain lasted for months, but Lolo would only use it for motivation to fuel the fire to overcome the hurdles to return to the Olympics.

The tripping over the last hurdle at the 2008 Olympics was attributed to a spinal problem where Lolo couldn't feel her feet. The doctor said the problem was that since she couldn't feel her feet; her brain wasn't able to process where her feet were. The surgery repaired a very painful tethered spinal cord.

With the surgery only a year before the 2012 Olympics, Lolo overcame the odds to come back and qualified for the 2012 Olympic team by placing third at the Olympic Trials. Lolo Jones came all the way back to make the Olympic 100-meter hurdle final again and finished fourth against an outstanding field.

Questions for Thought:

1. Lolo overcame a difficult childhood to be successful. How can you use her story for motivation?

2. Lolo thought about giving up track at one time, but her heart was still in it. How does heart factor into success?

3. Lolo overcame the odds to return to the Olympics. What odds have you overcome?

Jackie Joyner-Kersee: World's Greatest Female Athlete

Jackie Joyner-Kersee grew up in a violent neighborhood, witnessing murder and violence on the streets; however, her parents created an environment of love and a work ethic to achieve goals. Although drugs and alcohol surrounded her in her neighborhood, Jackie stayed away from that path and excelled in the classroom as an honor student. She began to show her promise as an athlete by long jumping over 17 feet when she was only 12 years old.

Jackie attended college at UCLA, but as an 18-year-old freshman, Jackie had to return home due to the tragic death of her 37-year-old mother, Mary, from a rare form of meningitis. Mary had been Jackie's inspiration and Jackie's grief threatened to derail her academic and athletic career. Jackie worked hard to perfect her skills and won the NCAA heptathlon two years in a row as well as the 1982 U.S. Championship. As Jackie prepared to compete in the 1983 World Championships in Helsinki, Finland, she pulled a hamstring and was forced to withdraw. She was also diagnosed with an asthmatic condition requiring constant medication, another challenge she would struggle with but consistently overcome.

In the 1984 Olympic Games in Los Angeles, California, Jackie had the lead in the heptathlon going into the final event, the 800 meters. However, her hamstring injury slowed her down and she ran less than a second too slow to win, with Glynis Nunn of Australia winning the gold by a margin of a mere five points. Jackie's career continued to soar as she tied the world record of 24-5 1/2 inches in the long jump.

At the 1988 Olympic Games, Jackie won gold medals in both the heptathlon and long jump. She also won a bronze medal in the long jump at the 1992 Olympic Games. The 1996 Olympic Games were held in Atlanta, Georgia, and Jackie had an opportunity to compete for gold in the heptathlon. Again, the recurrent hamstring injury re-appeared and forced her to withdraw from the heptathlon, but she still managed to win the Olympic bronze in the long jump.

Jackie Joyner-Kersee is known as one of the greatest female athletes of all time. Jackie won three gold, one silver, and two bronze medals over four consecutive Olympic Games, competing in the long jump and heptathlon events. She set world and Olympic records in the heptathlon and the long jump. Jackie's accomplishments serve as symbols of strength, courage, and hard work to achieve high goals.

Questions for Thought:

1. Jackie overcame a difficult environment growing up to be successful. What difficulties have you been able to overcome?

2. Asthma and injuries plagued Jackie, but she never gave up. What do you do when you feel like giving up?

3. Jackie stayed away from drugs and alcohol. What effect do you think drugs or alcohol would have on reaching your goals?

Chaunté Lowe: Flying High

When Chaunté Lowe was in sixth grade, she returned home from a track meet to find her family had lost their house. Her sisters had been sent to live with their father, who, trapped by drug addictions, spent most of his adult life in prison. Her mother struggled from her own addiction problems, and after they lost the house, Chaunté slept with her mother in rundown hotels and backs of cars. Chaunté was sent to live with an aunt, and eventually decided to live with her grandmother.

Embracing the sport of track and field was logical coming from a poverty standpoint. All it required was shorts and shoes. She was a sprinter, hurdler, and triple jumper, and made the national honor roll. She went on to Georgia Tech, where she became the school's first-ever female Olympian when she qualified for the 2004 Olympic Games in Athens as a sophomore.

In 2008, Chaunté and her husband, Mario, purchased their first home. With a new baby, she soon found out it's not easy for a new mother to remain competitive and was unable to earn money as an athlete. The economic crash of 2008 hit the couple hard. They purchased a rental property one day, and Mario lost his job the next. Both of their homes went into foreclosure. She and Mario moved into a tiny, one-bedroom apartment. Chaunté gave birth again, and this daughter had Asperger's syndrome.

Chaunté's Olympic performance had perhaps not yet matched her expectations in part because she was nursing children or recovering from childbirth. In 2004, she finished 13th in qualifying. In 2008, she placed sixth at the Beijing Olympics. In 2012, she went to the London Games as a favorite to medal, and again finished sixth. Chaunté had a tough 2015. She moved her training home base from Atlanta to Florida to obtain care for her special needs daughter.

Entering the Rio Games, Chaunté had cleared 6-7 at the U.S. Olympic Trials, the year's best mark in the world. Chaunté and three other jumpers were the only ones to make it to the final round of jumps. Chaunté was the final jumper. If she had cleared it, she would have won the gold. But she failed to do so and once again, she missed the podium by just one spot, finishing 4th.

Despite never earning an Olympic gold medal, Chaunté Lowe has been a great inspiration in the sport of track and field.

Questions For Thought:

1. Chaunté has made her family a priority. What are the important things in your life?

2. Chaunté has made four Olympic teams. What attributes does she possess that have led her to success?

3. Chaunté enjoys her high jumping and entertaining the crowd. She has fun with her sport. Do you have fun with your sport?

Sandi Morris: Flying Squirrel

Sandi Morris is nicknamed the "Flying Squirrel" because she leaps from high places on the track in pole vault and her personality has her jumping from hobby to hobby and always looking for an adventure.

Sandi won two South Carolina high school state championships and earned a scholarship to vault at the University of North Carolina. In her first year, Sandi was the only freshman to advance to indoor nationals and clear 14 feet. Her sophomore year, she struggled with the mental aspect of the sport and in the classroom. Though she was on the brink of making it to the 2012 Olympic Trials, she couldn't quite hit the qualifying standard.

Sandi transferred to Arkansas, where some of the best pole vaulters in NCAA history were. In 2015, Sandi broke the collegiate record at the second meet of the indoor season and jumped the current NCAA outdoor record at 15-5 ¾. She became a Bowerman semifinalist, a four-time All-American, a Nike athlete, and jumped for Team USA at the IAAF World Championships.

In May of 2016, Sandi snapped a pole and broke her left wrist at a meet in the Czech Republic. Seven weeks out from the Olympic Trials, she was able to run and train but couldn't vault for four weeks. At the Trials, she overcame the pain and finished second behind 2012 Olympic gold medalist Jenn Suhr.

On July 24, 2016, just days after the Trials, Sandi broke the outdoor American record at the American Track League meet in Houston. With a jump of 16-2, she scraped by Indoor World and American record-holder Jenn Suhr's previous outdoor record of 16-1 ½, set in 2006.

In Rio, Sandi missed her first attempts of 15-4 and 15-7, but cleared the heights on her second try, before missing three attempts at 16-0 ¾. Neither Morris nor Greece's Ekaterini Stefanidi cleared 16-0 ¾, but Stefanidi had one fewer miss than Sandi on the night, leaving Sandi with the silver medal.

With a silver medal on her plate and aiming for gold in four years, Sandi Morris went on to compete at the Brussels Diamond League meet after Rio. There, she shattered her outdoor American record when she cleared a height of 16-5 to win, making her only the second woman ever to clear 16-5 outdoors.

Questions for Thought:

1. Sandi Morris transferred to be surrounded by good vaulters. How do the people around you make you better?

2. How do you maintain your physical and mental condition when you are injured?

3. The pole vault requires a great amount of focus. How important is the skill of being able to focus well? How do you develop your ability to focus?

Louise Ritter: Overcoming Childhood Roadblocks

Louise Ritter's athletic career hit a roadblock at age 9 when she contracted rheumatic fever and was prohibited from any strenuous activity for almost three years. After her recovery, she established herself as a premier athlete, high jumping 5-11 1/2, the second highest high jump in the nation as a high school sophomore, in 1976.

When she enrolled at Texas Women's University in 1977, she was persuaded to change her style from the straddle to the Fosbury Flop, and her career soared to new heights. While attending Texas Woman's University, she captured national titles three out of four years and set her first American record at age 20. Louise held the American record on 10 different occasions, competed on three United States Olympic teams and was the premier women's high jumper in the United States for a decade from 1979 to 1989.

Despite her great success, her career was far from smooth sailing. Complications from injuries affected her jumping and she was forced to have arthroscopic knee surgery in 1983 and 1985, and in 1984 she injured her hip. Louise had a disappointing performance at the 1984 Olympics Games in Los Angeles, finishing eighth with a best jump of 6-3.

Entering the 1988 Olympic Games in Seoul, South Korea, the overwhelming favorite for the gold medal was world record holder Stefka Kostadinova of Bulgaria. Louise and Kostadinova were the only two jumpers to clear 6-7 in the competition and were tied for the lead. The bar went to 6-8 and they both missed all three attempts at that height. The rules in this situation call for a jump-off starting with one additional jump at the last height they both missed. Kostadinova missed her first jump of the jump-off and Louise followed by clearing the bar to equal her national record and secure the gold medal, becoming the first American woman to win a high jump gold medal in the Olympics in more than 50 years.

Questions for Thought:

1. Louise Ritter was prohibited for doing strenuous activity for three years. What would your life be like if you had to eliminate all strenuous activity?

2. Do you ever take your physical ability and the opportunities you have to engage in physical activities for granted?

3. Louise Ritter was a very successful athlete. How do you encourage others that may not be having as much success as you?

Ana Fidelia Quirot: I Will Run Again

Growing up, Ana Quirot had two heroes: Fidel Castro, the dictator of Cuba, and Cuban running legend Alberto Juantorena, who won gold medals in the 400- and 800-meter races at the 1976 Olympics. Ana was overweight as a girl, but lost weight when she began running seriously as a teen. At the age of 13, she was accepted into one of Cuba's prestigious state sports schools and began seriously training.

Ana found her niche in the 400 and 800 meters. Just as Ana was beginning to reach her peak performance years, the Cuban government decided to boycott the 1984 and 1988 Olympics Games. Ana's chance to prove herself on the international level came in the late 1980s and early 1990s. In 1989 she turned in an undefeated year in the 800-meter race. Her string of 39 consecutive victories in the 800 meters led to her being chosen as the I.A.A.F.'s female athlete of the year.

In the early weeks of a pregnancy, Ana ran the 800 meters in 1:56.80 for a bronze medal at the 1992 Summer Olympics in Barcelona, Spain. Ana was on top of the world, as she was widely admired for her beauty as well as her talent. In her seventh month of pregnancy, Ana was preparing to launder her clothes using a small kerosene-powered cook stove when an explosion occurred. In seconds, Ana was engulfed in a fire that burnt 38 percent of her body and brought her to the verge of death. She passed in and out of shock as her system reacted to the burns. Her baby, born prematurely, died. Scars on her face and neck marred her once-legendary beauty. When Ana regained consciousness in a hospital burn unit, Fidel Castro was standing at her bedside. "I will run again," she told him.

Ana faced a very lengthy recovery period, involving numerous skin-graft operations. To the amazement of medical experts, less than four months after the fire, she was back on the track. Ana's ability to move was restricted by the scar tissue on her stomach, arms, and hands. Her training time was restricted to the early morning and late evening hours when the sun could not hurt her damaged skin. Despite a scarred body, the fighting spirit of Ana Quirot still soared.

Ana was 29 years old when the accident occurred and was in the height of her career. She missed the 1994 track season due to a dozen rounds of plastic surgery. In 1995 she won the world championship at 800 meters, and the following year in the 1996 Olympic Games, she just missed winning the gold, capturing a silver medal. Ana Quirot's dramatic struggle to overcome adversity has turned her into a mythological hero in her own country.

Questions for Thought:

1. Despite being near death, Ana never gave up and overcame the odds. Think of a time you overcame the odds to accomplish a goal.

2. Ana was on top of the world until her accident. How do you think you would have reacted to the accident?

3. Ana recovered very quickly because of her positive attitude. How does attitude affect recovery?

Betty Robinson: First Female Olympic Gold Medalist

At age 16, American Betty Robinson competed in her first 100-meter race ever and finished second to the American record holder. In her second race ever, she equaled the world record for the 100 meters. Her third competition was the Olympic Trials, where she made the Olympic team. The 1928 Olympic Games was only her fourth competition, as she had only been running for four months.

The Amsterdam Olympics in 1928 was the first year that women were allowed to compete in the Olympic Games. Wearing a skirt, Betty lined up for the first women's Olympic final ever, the 100-meter dash. Betty sprinted to the win, equaling the world record and becoming the inaugural gold medal winner for women. She also added a silver medal as a member of the 4x100 meter relay team.

Tragedy struck in 1931 when Betty was severely injured in a plane crash. She was dragged from the wreckage with a severe concussion, a crushed arm, and a broken leg. A passerby mistook her for dead and drove her to the mortuary. Doctors gave her a slim chance of survival, let alone of walking again. She was in a coma for seven weeks, in a wheelchair for six months, and it took her two years before she could walk normally again.

While she was recuperating from her injuries, she missed an opportunity to compete before the home crowd at the 1932 Olympic Games in Los Angeles. With fierce determination, Betty battled back to make the 1936 Olympic team. Although unable to bend her knee for a crouching start in the 100 meters, she earned a spot running the third leg on the U.S. 4x100-meter relay team. The U.S. team was running behind the favored German team when the Germans dropped the baton and the U.S. went on to win.

For Betty Robinson, it was a remarkable rise, fall, and rise again; however, the damaged leg resulting from the crash robbed her of her peak years. But, by crossing the line first in Amsterdam years earlier, she guaranteed her place in the history books.

Questions for Thought:

1. Betty Robinson was a pioneer. Imagine what it would have felt like to be the very first person to win an Olympic gold medal.

2. How did Betty pave the way for future generations to come?

3. Betty struggled for years to return after injuries to compete again. What does that fierce determination say about a person? How do actions speak louder than words?

Brianna Rollins: From Rags to Rio

Her high school coach told her she could do it. She just had to believe it.

Brianna Rollins grew up with six younger brothers and her mother had a hard time landing jobs to earn money for her family. Sometimes they had no running water, no electricity, no food. Eventually, they had to move in with Brianna's grandparents. Nothing came easy for the Rollins', but with the help of her high school coach, friends, and relatives, Brianna slowly came to realize her potential as a person and an athlete.

Brianna was a scrawny ninth grader who had never competed in sports, so when she showed up in Miami Northwestern High track coach Carmen Jackson's office asking to join the track team, she had her doubts. She turned out to be a phenomenal athlete in high school, but struggled academically and lacked focus, easily distracted by boyfriends. Jackson set her straight. She helped her get her priorities in order and she signed with Clemson her senior year.

At Clemson, she grew homesick and lazy. She despised the cold and would quit workouts when she felt even a little pain. Once again, Jackson put her in her place—she told Brianna not to invite her to the pity party. And by her junior year in college, Brianna began to take things seriously on the track and in the classroom.

The 100-meter hurdles is one of the most competitive events in U.S. track and field. But after winning numerous conference titles, an NCAA indoor title as a sophomore at Clemson, and the NCAA outdoor title her senior year followed by breaking Gail Devers' 13-year-old U.S. record, Brianna made herself known in the hurdle world.

At the 2016 Olympic Trials at Hayward Field, nine women were ranked in the top 10 in the world in the 100-meter hurdles. But just three would make the Olympic team. Brianna was one of them as she won the gold.

In Rio, the US completed a first-ever 1-2-3 sweep in the event, with Brianna on top as the Olympic champion. Jackson had once told her she 'could break the world record, she could win the Olympics.' As Brianna Rollins crossed the finish line, her high school coach yelled "From rags to Rio!"

Questions for Thought:

1. Brianna originally struggled academically due to lack of focus but had a support system to get her on track. Who is your support system and how do they get you on track?

2. At one time Brianna considered herself lazy. What are the odds of success if you are not willing to work for it?

3. Is it possible to take a sport seriously and still have fun?

Wilma Rudolph: The Black Gazelle

Wilma Rudolph's race in life started very slowly as the 20th of 22 children. She was born prematurely and weighed only 4.5 pounds at birth. Because of racial segregation, Wilma and her mother were not permitted to be cared for at the local hospital because it was for whites only. The only black doctor was 50 miles away, which was a hardship on the Rudolph family's budget. Through the next several years, Wilma faced one hardship after another in the form of measles, mumps, scarlet fever, chicken pox, and double pneumonia.

When Wilma was 6 years old, it was discovered that her left leg and foot were becoming weak and deformed with polio, a crippling disease that had no cure. The doctor told Wilma that she would never walk again. Wilma and her mother were determined not to give up. With the help of the black medical college of Fisk University in Nashville, Wilma went through vigorous physical therapy using crutches, braces, and corrective shoes. Finally, by the age of 12, she could walk normally and decided to become an athlete.

In high school Wilma became a basketball star, setting state records for scoring and leading her team to the state championship. By the time she was 16, she earned a berth on the U.S. Olympic track and field team and came home from the 1956 Melbourne Games with an Olympic bronze medal in the 4x100 meter relay.

At the 1960 Summer Olympics in Rome, 80,000 spectators filled the Olympic Stadium in temperatures over 100 degrees. In the 100 meters, she tied the world record of 11.3 in the semifinals and then won the final in 11.0. However, because of a 2.75-meter per second wind, above the acceptable limit of two meters per second, she didn't receive credit for a world record. In the 200 meters, she broke the Olympic record in the opening heat in 23.2 and won the final in 24.0. In the 4x100-meter relay, Wilma, despite a poor baton pass, overtook Germany's anchor leg and the Americans, all women from Tennessee State, took the gold in 44.5 after setting a world record of 44.4 in the semifinals.

Wilma did more than promote her country. In her soft-spoken, gracious manner, she paved the way for future African American athletes, both men and women.

Questions for Thought:

1. Wilma Rudolph could not walk normally until she was 12, yet four years later, she was on the Olympic team. Do you ever think something is impossible?

2. Wilma was gracious and humble as an athlete. On a scale of 1-10 (10 high), how humble are you?

3. How does the Wilma Rudolph story inspire you?

REFERENCES

American Sport Education Program. (2008). *Coaching Youth Track and Field*. Champaign, IL: Human Kinetics.

Anderson, E. & Hibbert, A. (2006). *Training Games Coaching & Racing Creatively,* 4th ed. Mountain View, CA: TAFNews Press.

Athletics Canada. (2006). *Run, Jump, Throw- Teacher Resource*. Winnepeg, MB, Canada: Studio Publications.

Australian Sports Commission. *Athletics Play*. Melbourne, AUS.

Gozzoli, C., Simohamed, J., Malek, E., B. *IAAF Kid's Athletics- A Team Event for Children*.

International Association of Athletics Federation.

Jacoby, E. Fraley, B. (1995). *Complete Book of Jumps*. Champaign, IL: Human Kinetics. Karp, J. (2010). *101 Developmental Concepts and Workouts for Cross Country Runners*.

Monterey, CA: Coaches Choice.

New York Road Runners Club. (2014). *Track and Field Training Program*. http://www.nyrr.org

Pangrazi, R. (2001). *Dynamic Physical Education for Elementary School Children*. Boston, MA: Allyn and Bacon.

Peck, S. (2007). *101 Fun, Creative and Interactive Games for Kids*. Monterey, CA: Healthy Learning.

Quality Coaches, Quality Sports: National Standards for Sport Coaches, 2nd Edition. (2006). Reston, VA: NASPE National Association for Sport and Physical Education.

Stanbrough, M.E. (2012). *Motivational Moments in Men's Track and Field*. Emporia, KS: Roho Publishing.

---. (2012). *Motivational Moments in Women's Track and Field*. Emporia, KS: Roho Publishing.

---. (2014). *Running Games for Track and Field and Cross Country*. Emporia, KS: Roho Publishing.

---. (2015). *Track and Field Games*. Emporia, KS: Roho Publishing.

---. (2016). *Motivational Moments in 2016 Olympic Track and Field*. Emporia, KS: Roho Publishing.

USATF. (2000). *USA Track and Field Coaching Manual*. Champaign, IL: Human Kinetics.

Weiss, Howie. (2008). *Fun Fitness and Skills, The Powerful Original Games Approach*. Champaign, IL: Human Kinetics.

ABOUT THE AUTHOR

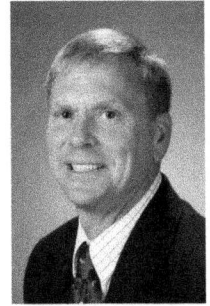

Dr. Mark Stanbrough is the head coach of the Emporia State University cross country team and is an assistant coach in track and field in charge of the middle distance and distance runners.

He is the Director of Coaching Education at Emporia State. ESU is one of only 12 universities in the nation that have been accredited by the National Committee for the Accreditation of Coaching Education. Besides coaching education courses, he teaches undergraduate and graduate courses in exercise physiology and sport psychology.

He is a national leader in coaching, currently serving as a board member on the National Committee for the Accreditation of Coaching Education. He was a co-founder of the first online course in HPER, which led to Emporia State HPER becoming the first physical education graduate program in the nation to offer a program completely online

Dr. Stanbrough has served as a head referee for USATF, NCAA, NAIA and Junior College national cross country and track and field championships. He is a member of the Emporia State University Athletic Hall of Honor and the Health, Physical Education, Recreation Hall of Honor and has won numerous coach-of-the-year awards at the high school and collegiate levels.

As the founder of Roho Publishing and Performance, which focuses on developing life skills for enhanced performance, Dr. Stanbrough has presented numerous presentations and workshops on coaching and mental skill development. He has worked with middle, high school, and collegiate teams in basketball, cross country, softball, tennis, track and field and volleyball in developing mental skills to enhance performance. Stanbrough has given over 200 presentations and authored 20 books on track and field, running, mental skills, and character development.

www.ingramcontent.com/pod-product-compliance
Lightning Source LLC
LaVergne TN
LVHW061343060426
835512LV00016B/2644